M000167348

A Handbook of
Traditional Chinese Dermatology

originally entitled
CHANG JIAN PI FU BING ZHONG YI ZHI LIAO JIAN BIAN

or

A Brief Compendium of the TCM Treatment of
Common Skin Diseases

by

LIANG JIAN-HUI

translated by

ZHANG TING-LIANG
&
BOB FLAWS

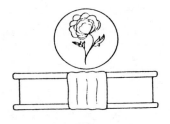

BLUE POPPY PRESS

Published by:

BLUE POPPY PRESS
1775 LINDEN AVE.
BOULDER, CO 80304

SECOND EDITION, MAY 1993

ISBN 0-936185-46-5

COPYRIGHT 1993 © BLUE POPPY PRESS

All rights reserved. No part of this book may be reproduced, stored in a retrieval system, or transcribed in any form or by any means, electronic, mechanical, photocopy, recording, or any other means, without the prior written permission of the publisher.

The information in this book is given in good faith. However, the translators and the publisher cannot be held responsible for any error or omission. Nor can they be held in any way responsible for treatment given on the basis of information contained in this book. The publisher make this information available to English language readers for scholarly and research purposes only.

The publishers do not advocate nor endorse self-medication by laypersons. Chinese medicine is a professional medicine. Laypersons interested in availing themselves of the treatments described in this book should seek out a qualified professional practitioner of Chinese medicine.

Printed at Westview Press, Boulder, CO on acid free, recycled paper.

10 9 8 7 6 5 4

recycled paper

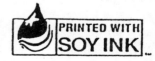

Translators' Preface to Second Edition _____

A Handbook of Traditional Chinese Dermatology is a functional or denotative translation of *Chang Jian Pi Fu Bing Zheng Yi Zhi Liao Jian Bian (A Brief Compendium of the Chinese Medical Treatment of Common Skin Diseases)* by Liang Jian-hui of the Dermatology Department of the Guangdong Provincial TCM Hospital. It was originally published in Chinese by the People's Hygiene Press in 1986. It has been translated by Zhang Ting-liang and myself as the third of a series of joint translations of TCM clinical manuals. The present volume is the second edition of this translation and we have taken the opportunity to make numerous corrections and improvements in this edition. We have changed much of the terminology to conform more closely to Nigel Wiseman's in *A Glossary of Chinese Medical Terms and Acupuncture Points* and also to render the translation more accurate; we have corrected some of our pharmacological nomenclature; and we have added Pinyin identifications for the medicinals which appear in the formulas and formula appendix. Because of this, we have deleted the previous index of medicinal ingredients with their Chinese characters.

As Dr. Liang points out in the opening to this book, classically, dermatology was not an independent specialty in Traditional Chinese Medicine. Rather, what is now referred to as *pi fu ke* or dermatology was a part of *wai ke*. In general, Chinese medicine can be divided into two broad divisions, *nei ke* or internal medicine and *wai ke* or external medicine. *Wai ke* means the diagnosis and treatment of diseases manifesting on the exterior portions of the body. In Chinese medicine, the tissues that make up the *wai* or exterior are the *pi mao*, skin and hair, *ji rou*, muscles and flesh, and *jin gu*, sinews and bones.[1] Traditionally, *wai ke* included traumatology (*shang ke* or *die da ke*), dermatology (*pi fu ke*), orthopedics (*zheng gu ke*), and surgery (*shou zhu*).

The contemporary tendency to translate *wai ke* simply as surgery blurs the traditional Chinese meaning and logic of this term. Till now, most English language texts for practitioners of TCM have concentrated on *nei ke* or internal medicine. However, in order to understand and appreciate Traditional Chinese Medicine as a complete system of medicine and in order to practice Chinese medicine as a clinician, an understanding of *wai ke* is of fundamental importance.

Our decision to translate and publish this book was motivated in large part by my own frustration in treating dermatological conditions. These have been some of the most frustrating and recalcitrant conditions I have been called upon to treat. In discussing my own experience with other American practitioners of TCM, I have come to the conclusion that I am not alone in finding dermatologic conditions difficult to treat. Part of this difficulty has been simply incomplete literature on the diagnosis and treatment of dermatologic conditions by Chinese medicine. It is our hope that the publishing of this book will help fill that gap and enable more American practitioners of TCM to treat dermatologic conditions from a more informed position.

Often the difference between success or failure in the treatment of dermatologic conditions depends on their proper external treatment. Without such external therapy, acupuncture and internal medication are often so slow in effecting appreciable change that the patient loses faith and patience and therefore aborts the treatment prematurely. This is bad for the patient, since, ultimately, they are left with the disease. This is bad for the practitioner since they will not get referrals from such patients. And this is bad for Chinese medicine in

---

[1] The *nei* or interior is made up of the *zang fu* or viscera and bowels, while the *jing luo*, the channels and connecting vessels communicate between the *nei* and *wai*.

America since patients, both actual and potential, and other healthcare professionals may assume that since treatment for such conditions was not successful, Chinese medicine in general is ineffective or suspect. This book contains many external treatments which can be combined with internal medication or acupuncture. Those of which I have had occasion to use have proven effective when correct differential diagnosis has been made.

Western practitioners of Traditional Chinese Medicine may be surprised at how much modern Western medicine this book contains. As a recent Chinese publication, this book exemplifies the contemporary Chinese endeavor to and penchant for combining traditional Chinese and modern Western medicines. In the original text, under the headings "Pathogenesis and Pathophysiology", both traditional Chinese and modern Western theories concerning the etiology of each disease are given. We have been careful in this translation to distinguish between these two levels of discourse. In translating the Western medical terminology, we have tried to adopt the standards of *The Merck Manual* as far as was possible. I believe we were quite fortunate since Zhang Ting-liang had worked for several years on a Chinese — Japanese — English medical dictionary before coming to America. For Western practitioners of Traditional Chinese Medicine who are unfamiliar with Western (*i.e.* Latin/Greek) medical terminology, we have appended a glossary of technical dermatological terms.

Although this is one of the most complete English language texts on the TCM diagnosis and treatment of dermatological disease, we caution practitioners that is should only be used as a jumping off point. In fact, it is not exhaustive and categorically definitive. For instance, the present text only lists the yang vacuity *zheng* or pattern of disharmony for scleroderma when, in fact, a yin vacuity pattern also exists based on the Chinese literature and my personal clinical experience. Therefore, practitioners still must do a TCM diagnosis based on a discrimination of patterns of disharmony (*bian zheng*) and parse out each individual patient's diagnosis. For this purpose, "The Main Concepts of the Pathophysiology of Skin Diseases", "Various (TCM) Patterns

Associated with Dermatological Diseases", and "Internal Treatment Methods for Dermatological Diseases" are invaluable sections.

The two other English language books on TCM dermatology of which I am aware are: *Clinic of Traditional Chinese Medicine (II)*, part of the Shanghai College of TCM Publishing House's *Practical English-Chinese Library of Traditional Chinese Medicine* and *The English-Chinese Encyclopedia of Practical Traditional Chinese Medicine, Vol. 16, Dermatology*. I also recommend practitioners to cross-check the diagnoses and treatments in these two books as well. No one book on any clinical specialty is categorically complete.

However, above all, my personal advice is to work out each patient's diagnosis step by step and piece by piece based upon their signs, symptoms, tongue, and pulse, paying special attention to the specific nature of the lesions themselves, and then, treat for *your* diagnosis, regardless of what this book or similar books say should be the diagnosis. In other words, play what you see. For me, this is one of the cardinal rules of the practice of Chinese medicine. This is especially the case since, frequently, Western patients do not display the same patterns as Chinese with the same frequency.

As an extension of this, it is very important that whatever formulas are given in this or other such books be modified to fit the individual needs of specific patients. In Chinese, *jia jian* means additions and subtractions. In clinical practice, the vast majority of prescriptions written contain these two words. This means that, although a guiding prescription has been selected as the basis of the prescription, certain ingredients have been left out and others have been added based upon an understanding of the individual diagnosis, the pathophysiology of the case, and on the presenting signs and symptoms as *biao* or branches.

In order to understand how to modify a given formula, one must first have a carefully worked out, individualized diagnosis and then must understand the natures and uses of the individual ingredients in a formula and their synergism. This type of proficiency in writing individual prescriptions is usually learned in a course called in Chinese TCM colleges *fang ji xue* or the study of prescriptions. In such colleges, the study of prescriptions and prescription writing and modification come before the study of individual specialties such as dermatology.

We have based our pharmacological identifications on the *Zhong Yao Da Ci Dian (Encyclopedia of Chinese Materia Medica)*, Bensky and Gamble's *Chinese Herbal Medicine: Materia Medica*, Hong-yen Hsu's *Oriental Materia Medica: A Concise Guide*, *A Barefoot Doctor's Manual*, and Stuart and Read's *Chinese Materia Medica*. Medicinals are first identified by Latin pharmacological nomenclature followed by PinYin in parentheses.

Appendix I is an intrinsic part of the original Chinese edition of this work. It is a compilation of the standard dermatological prescriptions referred to in the text with their ingredients. Formulas which appear in the text followed by a numeral in parentheses are arranged numerically in Appendix I. Appendix II is a glossary of Western medical dermatological terms. These terms have been used in this translation because of their professional precision. By and large, they are descriptive terms which lack any bias inherent in Western medicine.

Zhang Ting-liang and myself hope that this book will contribute to raising the standards of the American practice of Traditional Chinese Medicine in the West in general, and, in particular, of TCM dermatology. We also hope that it will help alleviate skin diseases which are so emotionally painful for their sufferers because they are unsightly and disfiguring. And further, we hope that this revised edition will make the material contained herein more useful and more in line with standards of translation which have emerged within our profession since this book's first publication in 1988.

Bob Flaws
April 19, 1993

Contents _____

Part Two

The Treatment of Common Dermatological Diseases, 17

One: Eczema & Dermatitis, 17

Two: Urticarias, 33

Three: Suppurative Dermatitis, 37

Part One

Outline of the Differentiation & Treatment of Dermatological Diseases

Dermatological diseases refer to disorders of the skin and its appendages. In ancient China, dermatology was a part of *wai ke*.[1] Therefore, there are no existing (classical) systematic works (specifically) on dermatology. *Wai ke* includes skin diseases because the skin is the most external layer of the body. Because of this, most information concerning skin disease is found mixed (in with non-dermatological information) in *wai ke* texts.

As early as the 14th century BCE, the word *jie* (scabious rash) was used in inscriptions on bones and tortoise shells. In the Zhou dynasty (11th century BCE), *shi yi* (dietary medicine), *ji yi* (internal medicine), *yang yi* (surgery), and *shou yi* (veterinary medicine) had become separate medical specialties. *Yang yi* means traditional Chinese surgery in which skin diseases are included. The *Huang Di Nei Jing* includes passages concerning the causes of skin disease. In *Prescriptions for Emergency* by Ge Hong (341 CE) are recorded many effective methods used for the treatment of skin diseases. The pathogenesis and pathophysiology of skin diseases are extensively expounded upon in *The General Treatise on the Cause and Symptoms of Disease* written by Cao Yuan-fang in 610 CE. Furthermore, detailed descriptions of the treatment of various kinds of skin diseases

---

[1] *Wai ke* means specialty in (diseases occurring in) the outside (of the body). The *wai* or outside is comprised of the skin and hair, muscles and flesh, sinews and bones. The *nei* or inside is composed of the viscera and bowels, while the channels and connecting vessels connect the inside with the outside.

1

are recorded in *A Thousand Golden Prescriptions* by Sun Si-miao in 652 and in *Essential Points of Wai Ke* by Chen Zi-ming in 1263. Other classics dealing with skin diseases include *The Main Points for Wai Ke* by Qi De-zhi in 1335, *The Orthodox Manual of Wai Ke* by Chen She-gong in 1617, and *The Golden Mirror of Ancestral Medicine* by Wu Qian in 1742.

Traditional Chinese Medicine has made great contributions to the (development) of dermatological science. Many therapeutic methods based on the application of (one or more) ingredients (now used throughout the world) originated in China. For instance, Sulphur was used to treat scabies long before the time of Christ. Mercury was also first used in treating skin diseases in China. Other innovative usages include the oil of Semen Hydnocarpi for leprosy and Arsenic preparations for syphilis.

Skin diseases are among the most common diseases of the people. Traditional Chinese Medicine is renowned for its rich experience in treating dermatological disorders of all kinds through its application of its (principles of) differentiation and treatment. As in other (Chinese medical) specialties, (these principles and therapeutic methods) are based on the fundamental theories of Traditional Chinese Medicine. Since different stages of a single disease may manifest similarly, therefore, (in Chinese Medicine) one may use different therapies to treat the same disease and similar therapies to treat different diseases as long as they present similar symptoms.

2

One

The Main Concepts of Pathophysiology in Dermatology

Traditional Chinese Medicine believes that the human body is an integral whole in which the skin and muscles and the five *zang* (organs) and six *fu* (bowels) are interrelated interiorly and exteriorly by the channels and connecting vessels. Therefore, the four methods of diagnosis and the eight principles of differentiation can never be over-emphasized in discriminating the nature of a disease. Also, the treatment of the internal cause of a disease should not be neglected when treating external symptoms.

In ancient Chinese medical literature, all kinds of skin lesions are called *chuang*. *The Golden Mirror of Ancestral Medicine* says "Gangrene develops from the tendons and bones of yin nature. Carbuncles are rooted in the flesh of yang nature. (Whereas) ulcers originate from between the skin and the flesh. *Chuang* is a synonym for lesions which take root in the skin." This quotation implies that *chuang* are superficial conditions, such as syphilis, eczema, scabies, multiform erythema, dermatosis due to lacquer allergy, infantile eczema, and thrush.

The *Huang Di Nei Jing* states that "pain, itching, and *chuang* of all kinds are ascribed to the heart." The heart governs fire and heat. Fire is an extreme form of heat and heat is a mild form of fire. When heat is extreme, *chuang* are painful. When heat is not extreme, *chuang* itch. Moreover, according to *The General Treatise on the Cause and Symptoms of Disease*, "The lungs govern the qi and are connected with the skin and hair. The spleen controls the muscle. Qi vacuity leaves the skin loose and the pores open, therefore leaving one susceptible to attack by wind and dampness. Internal heat makes the spleen qi warm. This warm spleen qi gives rise to warm earth in the muscles. The combination of dampness and heat thus cause carbuncles and furuncles to arise on the face and over the rest of the body."

Clinically, acute dermatological conditions, such as swelling, ulceration, the discharge of pus, inflammation, itching, watery blisters, and pustules, are mostly related to the invasion of wind, dampness, and heat. Most often, these symptoms are also associated with excesses of the heart, lungs, and spleen. On the other hand, dry skin, scaling, pigment sedimentation, and hair loss are due to vacuity and exhaustion of *ying* blood. These symptoms are related to vacuity of the liver and kidney and are vacuous in nature. In addition, insects and blood stagnation are responsible for a number of skin diseases.

Two

Various (TCM) Patterns Associated With Dermatological Diseases

All skin diseases cause certain damage to the skin and it is often the morphology of this damage which serves as the basis of differentiation. As a rule, watery lesions are mostly due to damp heat. Suppurative lesions are due to heat toxins. Leukoderma is due to qi stagnation. Erythema is due to blood heat. Purplish spots are due to blood stagnation, and papules are due to wind heat. Reddish wheals are often ascribed to wind heat; while white ones are ascribed to wind cold. Bloody scabs are related to the existence of heat toxin; while ulcerations are due to damp heat. Scaling in acute dermatological diseases implies the existence of remnant heat, while scaling in chronic diseases is due to blood vacuity and wind dryness. Remarkable scratches suggest a predominance of wind. Rhagas is suggestive of cold or dryness. Numerous nodulations are indicative of stagnation of qi and blood. The early stage is due to blood vacuity.

For convenience of differentiation and treatment, the clinical manifestations of skin disease are typically grouped into eight patterns: wind, cold, summer heat, dampness, dryness, fire, insects, and blood stasis. Some books also list the categories blood vacuity, Insufficiency of the liver and kidneys, and toxins. However, these last three groups are covered by the former eight patterns. wind due to blood vacuity is still wind. dryness due to blood vacuity is still dryness. Insufficiency of liver kidney yin manifests as blood vacuity and therefore evolves into wind and dryness. And insufficiency of liver and kidney yang also presents as wind. So-called toxin evil, refers to chemical and food allergies as well as to lacquer allergy.

However, all these manifest as wind and fire.

The specific features of these eight patterns are as follows:

1. Wind Pattern

Wind evil can be subdivided into internal and external wind. External wind suggests that the condition is caused by factors from the outside world. Internal wind is often generated by yin vacuity of the liver and kidney and insufficiency of the yin and blood. Wind pattern is often marked by papules and wheals which are characterized by their mobility all over the body and their extreme itchiness. The patient tends to scratch until they bleed. In this case, scabs form quickly and there is seldom infection or suppuration since the situation is dry in nature. The tongue body is typically red with a thin, white coating. The pulse is taut. It is easy to distinguish external wind because of its migrating nature. Thus the saying, "Wind is characterized by its mobility and unexpected changeability." On the other hand, skin diseases caused by internal wind are all due to vacuity of yin and blood and are therefore characterized by dryness.

2. Cold Pattern

Cold is likewise subdivided into external and internal cold. External cold here refers to those symptoms due to invasion by external pathogens. Where internal cold refers to those symptoms reflecting functional deterioration and insufficiency of yang qi. Either may present as wheals or rashes. However, the color of the affected area tends to be pale, pink, or dark purple. The surface of the skin feels smooth and may lack elasticity. Other accompanying symptoms include nausea, lumbar soreness, hair loss, loose teeth, cold limbs, or water stools. In females, there may be accompanying irregular menstruation. In males, there may be spermatorrhea or impotence. (In such cases, typically) the course of the disease is long. The tongue coating is often thin and white and the pulse is thready and slow.

3. Summer Heat Pattern

(As the name implies, this pattern) is characterized by the season. Diseases occurring before *xia zhi* (summer solstice) are called *bing wen* (warm diseases); while those occurring after *xia zhi* are called *bing shu* (summer heat diseases). This (latter) condition happens mostly during the heat of summer due to exposure to pathogenic heat. It is marked by the sudden onset of papules, erythema, watery blisters, and pustules. Accompanying symptoms often include fever, thirst, dark and short urination, a scarlet tongue body proper with a yellow, sticky or yellow, thick coating, and a superficial, rapid or slippery, rapid pulse.

4. Dampness Pattern

(This pattern) is again subdivided into external and internal dampness. External dampness refers to those symptoms caused by heat derived from stagnant dampness due to retention of water dampness. This, in turn, is due to dysfunction of the spleen in transforming and transporting. It is recorded in the *Huang Di Nei Jing* that, "All cases of swelling and puffiness due to dampness are ascribed to the spleen." Papules, watery blisters, pustules, ulcerations, discharge of serous fluid, puffiness and discharge of yellowish fluid may all be present. (Dampness) may also cause extreme formication and may take a protracted course. Nausea, malaise, and a low fever may all be present. The tongue body proper is light red with a white, sticky or yellow, sticky coating. The pulse is slow.

5. Dryness Pattern

Dryness is also subdivided into external and internal dryness. External pathogens refer to such natural (environmental) causes as dry weather in the autumn. Internal dryness originates from insufficiency of body fluids or insufficiency of blood. The common symptoms of this category of skin disease are dry skin, desquamation, rhagas, and lichenification. Subjective symptoms may include itching but (this pattern) is seldom accompanied by ulceration. The disease may have a long course since most cases (of dryness) are chronic. Other symptoms may include thirst and disturbed sleep. The tongue is red with a white, dry coating. The pulse is wiry.

6. Fire Pattern

Similar to heat, (fire is likewise) characterized by Hot symptoms. The difference (between these two) lies only in the severity of the pattern. fire pattern can either be caused by external fire pathogens or the hyperactivity of fire in the internal organs. Common local signs and symptoms are redness, swelling, heat, pain, and itching. Erythema of varied size and densely packed papules or watery blisters are common. All these symptoms may be accompanied by fever, constipation, and short, red urination. The tongue body proper is red or even scarlet with a dry, yellowish coating. The pulse is full and rapid or slippery and rapid.

7. Skin diseases caused by insect bite

This category of disease is mostly caused by insect sting or contact with insects. These give rise to papules, vesicles, pustules, and erythema or wheals. (This condition is characterized by) its aggressive expansion or discharge of yellowish fluid. The itching sensation is extreme, as if a worm were crawling (on one). (Such diseases) are most often infectious, (viz. scabies, crabs, lice, fleas, etc.).

8. Blood Stagnation Pattern

This condition involves the obstruction of the blood vessels and the impaired circulation of qi and blood. Its common symptoms are increase of pigmentation, (the appearance of) purple spots, dark red nodulations, or subcutaneous nodulations. Skin lesions are typically localized and symptoms are recalcitrant to treatment over a protracted disease course. The tongue body proper may be dark red or purplish with a yellow, thick coating. The pulse is wiry or hesitant.

Three _____

Internal Treatment of Dermatological Diseases

1. Expelling Wind

A. Expelling wind and enriching the blood: This method is indicated in those conditions caused by internal wind due to blood vacuity which manifests as insufficiency of yin and blood simultaneously. *Gui Zhi Dang Gui Tang* (1) with modifications is often applicable for skin diseases of dry nature with copious scaling, such as ichthyosis and psoriasis during their static and degenerative stages.

B. Expelling wind and consolidating the surface: This method is indicated for skin diseases caused by wind invasion due to vacuity of the superficial regions of the body. The main symptom is aversion to wind. Most cases are marked by their chronic recurrence. (For this,) *Yu Ping Feng San* (2) with modifications is often employed in the treatment of chronic allergic skin diseases, such as chronic urticaria.

C. Expelling wind and causing perspiration: This method is often used in cases of superficial and replete nature due to exposure to wind pathogens. *Xiao Feng San* (3) is often employed for the treatment of acute allergic conditions like acute urticaria and acute dermatitis.

2. Dispersing Cold

A. Warming the channels and scattering cold: This method is often applied in the treatment of those conditions caused by obstruction of the channels and connecting vessels due to attack by external cold

9

pathogens. For this purpose, *Dang Gui Si Ni Tang* (4) is indicated. (This formula) is frequently used for conditions relating to impeded blood circulation, such as frostbite.

B. Dispersing cold and strengthening yang: This method is often applied in those skin diseases resulting from obstruction of the channels and connecting vessels due to insufficiency of yang and qi and degeneration of the internal organs. *Yang He Tang* (5) is one example of a commonly used formula for chronic skin disorders involving impeded blood circulation, such as scleroderma.

3. Clearing Summer Heat

A. Clearing heat and eliminating dampness: This method is often employed for the treatment of those conditions due to the presence of dampness in turn due to exposure to heat pathogens. *Qing Hao Yi Ren Tang* (6) is advised for the treatment of summer-time skin diseases, such as summer dermatitis.

B. Clearing heat and resolving toxins: This method is recommended for the treatment of suppurative conditions in the summer, such as furuncles, boils, and impetigo, for which *Qing Shu Tang* (7) (is indicated).

4. Eliminating Dampness

A. Eliminating dampness and clearing heat: This method is often applied in the treatment of those conditions with profuse fluid discharge because of heat derived from stagnant dampness. *Bi Xie Shen Shi Tang* (8) may be employed to treat acute eczema and contact dermatitis.

B. Eliminating dampness and fortifying the spleen: This method is indicated for those skin diseases due to spleen vacuity causing dysfunction in the transmission of water dampness. *Jian Pi Shen Shi Tang* (9) may be used for allergic skin diseases which are associated with poor body constitution, such as infantile eczema and chronic pediatric urticaria.

5. Moistening Dryness

A. Moistening dryness and replenishing the blood: This method is desirable for the treatment of those conditions due to wind and dryness in turn due to blood vacuity complicated by yin vacuity. *Di Huang Yin* (10) is indicated for chronic, itching dermatitis, such as chronic eczema and neurodermatitis.

B. Moistening dryness and promoting the production of fluids: This method is indicated for the treatment (of skin diseases) due to Insufficiency of body fluid. *Run Fu Tang* (11) is often applied to treat dry, itching dermatitis, such as common dermatitis.

6. Purgation of Fire

A. Discharging fire and resolving toxins: This method is indicated for symptoms due to exposure to fire toxins marked by acute and infectious lesions. *Wu Wei Xiao Du Yin* (12) is often used to treat acute, suppurative disorders such as sever cases of systemic pustules, furuncles, and boils.

B. Discharging fire and cooling the blood: This method is indicated for those conditions caused by hyperactivity of fire of the internal organs which are often marked by symptoms of hot blood. This typically manifests as extensive erythema with severe systemic symptoms. *Sheng Di Yin Hua Tang* (13) is an example of an often employed formula for the treatment of redness, swelling, heat, and pain of an acute nature, such as dermatitis due to exposure to lacquer.

7. Dispelling Stasis

A. Dispelling stasis and cooling the blood: This method is indicated

11

for those conditions due to retention of stagnant blood and obstruction by hot blood manifesting as erythema and nodulation. *Liang Xue Si Wi Tang* (14) is frequently used in the treatment of telangiactasic, erythemic, and histo-progressive psoriasis.

B. Dispelling stasis and activating the blood: This method is recommended for the treatment of dermatologic diseases caused by retention of stagnant blood due to obstructed blood and qi circulation. *Bu Yang Huan Wu Tang* (15) is the preferred treatment for nodular painful skin diseases, such as nodular erythema and panniculitis.

Four _____

External Therapies for Dermatological Diseases

1. Herbal Medicines (*Cao Yao*)

Macerated fresh medicinal herbs are often applied topically or the juice of these herbs is used as a lotion since certain fresh herbs can stop itching, dispel inflammation, kill bacteria, and cleanse turbidity. For example, the juice of fresh Herba Violae Yedoensis (*Zi Hua Di Ding*) may be used externally for pustules. Macerated Herba Portulacae Oleraceae (*Ma Chi Xian*) may be applied directly to swellings due to boils. And macerated Herba Tougucao (*Tou Gu Cao*) may be applied externally to tinea pedis.

2. Pastes (*Gao Yao*)

(Herbal pastes) are noted not only for their effect in activating the Blood by removing stagnation but also for relieving swelling, stopping pain, and resolving nodulation. They are frequently used because they can prevent the affected surface from being infected by various bacteria. The most commonly used pastes are *Qian Chui Gao* (16) and *Tai Yi Gao* (17). However, pastes should not be applied if there is production of serous fluid. Zhou Yue pointed out in his *Personal Experience in Wai Ke* (1838) that, "Pastes are contraindicated when damp heat toxins exist on the lower extremities. (If misused,) the confined heat will move transversely and spread even more extensively. Pastes are advisable in protracted cases." This quotation indicates that the application of pastes in cases of profuse fluid discharge will impede the drainage of pus.

3. Resolvants (*Wei Fu Yao*)

These powdered medicines, for example *Huang Jin San* (18) and *Si Huang San* (19), are characterized by their ability to dispel inflammation, stop pain, dispel swelling, and their ability to disperse heat. Shen Dou-huan, in his Revealing the *Mystery of Wai Ke* (1604), said, "(The purpose of) employing resolvants is to resolve and disperse the existing toxins (possible) accumulation and growth."

4. Ointments (*Yuan Gao*)

Ointments are also called *You Gao* (oil-based ointments). *Qing Dai Gao* (20), *Si Huang Gao* (19), *Sheng Ji Gao* (21), and *Run Ji Gao* (22), are often used to stop itching, dispel inflammation, and clear and cleanse turbidity. However, ointments are also contraindicated in cases where there is profuse serous discharge.

5. Tinctures (*Ding Ji*)

Tinctures, (in Chinese) called "wines", are able to stop itching, dispel inflammation, and kill bacteria. The most commonly used (dermatological) tinctures are *Bai Xie Feng Ding* (23), *Hong Ling Jiu* (24), and *Zhi Yang Ding* (25).

6. Powders (*Fen Ji*)

Powders are also called medicated mixtures, such as *Qing Dai San* (20) and *Yu Lu San* (26). They are known not only for their drying and protective properties but also for their ability to clear heat.

7. Extracts (*You Ji*)

Extracts are also called medicated oils. *Gan Cao You* (27), for example, is often used to moisten the skin, stop itching, disperse inflammation, and to clear and cleanse turbidity.

8. Washes (*Shui Fen Ji*)

San Huang Xi Ji (28) and *Dian Dao San Xi Ji* (29) are often used because of their dispersing inflammation, stopping itching, clearing heat, drying, and protective properties.

9. Wet Compresses (*Shi Fu*)

Compresses made with medicated water can be used for clearing hat, dispersing inflammation, and clearing and cleansing turbidity. For instance, a medicated water (suitable for use as a compress) can be made from Cortex Phellodendri (*Huang Bai*), Radix Glycyrrhizae (*Gan Cao*), Radix Sophorae Flavescentis (*Ku Shen*), and Fructus Cnidii Monnieri (*She Chuang Zi*).

10. Medicinal baths (*Yao Yu*)

Besides dispersing inflammation, stopping itching, and killing bacteria, medicinal baths also facilitate the healing of exfoliative keratolysis. *Ku Shen Tang* (30) and *Yin Xie Bing Yu Ji* are most commonly used (for these purposes). It is recorded in *Revealing the Mystery of Wai Ke* that, "It is advisable to bathe or steam swellings due to skin conditions of all kinds with medicated water for the first one or two days in order to reopen the striae of the skin and to restore regular and harmonious blood circulation. By relieving possible occlusion of the minute pores, (this method) frees the patient from later distress and also disperses toxins."

11. Fumigation (*Yan Xun Liao Fa*)

Fumigation is used to stop itching and kill bacteria. (It is often used in cases of) chronic eczema, neurodermatitis, and tinea of the hand. It is pointed out in *Revealing the Mystery of Wai Ke* that, "For long term ulceration on the shanks, tenacious tinea, and scabies of all kinds showing no sign of improvement after continuous treatment, try fumigation therapy by igniting a mixtures of ingredients. This method will facilitate the healing process."

12. Moxibustion (*Ai Jiu*)

The direct application of heat from an ignited moxa stick can be used to destroy the lesion, such as in the treatment of common warts.

13. Cupping (*Ba Guan*)

(Cupping) is used to suck out toxins as in cases of wasp sting and centipede bite.

14. Body Needles (*Ti Zhen*), Ear Needles (*Er Zhen*), and Plum Blossom Needles (*Mei Hua Zhen*)

Needles can be used to directly stimulate the affected area. For instance, clavus can be treated with acupuncture. Alopecia areata and neurodermatitis can be treated by plum blossom needling. (In addition,) acupuncture and auricular acupuncture are frequently used to adjust the physiological functions of the body so as to achieve the therapeutic effect. Examples are the treatment of urticaria, pruritus, and flat warts with acupuncture or auricular acupuncture.

Part Two

The Treatment of Common Dermatological Diseases

One

Eczema & Dermatitis

1. Plant and Contact Dermatitis
Yao Wu Jie Chu Xing Pi Wan

Pathogenesis and pathophysiology: Called *gao yao feng* (herbal plaster wind) in ancient times and, due to incompatibility with the body and infirmity of the striae of the skin, contact with certain plants or externally used chemicals may cause inflammation of the skin.

Diagnosis: Having been exposed to externally used chemicals, lesions with well-defined margins suddenly appear in the areas of contact. Erythema, papules, water blisters, even necrosis may present. (The patient) may complain of itching, burning, or pain in severe cases.

Treatment

Internal Medication:

Xiao Feng San (3) with modifications is recommended for the purpose of activating the blood, dispelling wind, and eliminating dampness.

External Therapies:

1) A cold compress may be made from a decoction of Radix Glycyrrhizae (*Gan Cao*), Cortex Phellodendri (*Huang Bai*), Radix Sanguisorbae (*Di Yu*), Radix Sophorae Flavescentis (*Ku Shen*), and Radix Et Rhizoma Rhei (*Da Huang*), 30g each.

2) Prepared Gypsum Fibrosum (*Shi Gao*), prepared Talcum (*Hua Shi*), and prepared Hallyositum Rubrum (*Chi Shi Zhi*), 500g @, plus prepared Calamina (*Lu Gan Shi*), 250g. Grind the above into a fine powder, mix into a paste with sesame oil, and apply externally.

3) *San Huang Xi Ji* (28) may be used as a lotion.

2. Saliva Dermatitis
Kou Shui Xing Pi Yan

Pathogenesis and pathophysiology: This condition is also called *tian zhui chuang* (licking lesion). Babies may develop a habit of moistening their lips with their tongue because of being dry. This may result in long-term irritation by saliva and habitual rubbing with their hands.

Diagnosis: This problem mostly affects children from three to ten years of age. It is characterized by moist erythema around the lips. If the patient is wearing long sleeves, saliva-like paste may be noted on the sleeves.

Treatment

Most cases do not require internal administration of medicine. Either a 1% berberine ointment or powdered Rhizoma Coptidis Chinensis (*Huang Lian*) mixed with sesame oil may be applied to the lips. The patient will thus abandon their habit due to the bitter taste. These herbs also dispel inflammation and moisten the skin.

3. Diaper Rash
Niao Bu Pi Yan

Pathogenesis and pathophysiology: This condition is called "red buttocks" in the classics. Quite often the thighs of the baby may be red and abraded due to the constant friction of wet diapers against the skin. (According to modern Western medicine) diaper rash is caused by ammonia derived from urea decomposed by gram positive bacillus. In *Revealing the Mystery of Wai Ke* it is said, "Diaper rash may start in the first month after birth. As both the upper and lower limbs of the infant are bound, the areas underneath the chin, armpits, and groin are most likely to be attacked by damp heat which frequently leads to ulceration. The mother is to be blamed for her negligence."

Diagnosis: At first the affected area is reddish and rough with tiny scales. Maculopapules or vesicles are commonly seen. Sometimes, pinhead-like pustules or fluid discharge and ulceration in severe cases may also be seen. The affected area, although at first restricted to the area covered by the diaper, may spread to the lower abdomen and thigh.

Treatment

1) For fluid discharge: use a wet compress made from a 5% solution of Radix Glycyrrhizae (*Gan Cao*).

2) Reddish papules: dust (affected area) with *Fu Fang Ku Shen Feng* (33).

3) Apply *Hong Tang You Gao* (34) externally to the affected area.

4) (According to) *Revealing The Mystery of Wai Ke*: "Dust the affected area with a finely ground powder of Terra Flava Usta (*Fu Long Gan*). Cover with paper and it will heal soon."

4. Lacquer Rash
Qi Xing Pi Yan

Pathogenesis and pathophysiology: The classic name of dermatitis rhus

19

is "lacquer lesion". (Some people are) born allergic to lacquer. They are easily affected whenever they come into contact with lacquer fluid, lacquer trees, lacquerware, or lacquer toxins due to the uncompactness of the striae of their skin. In modern times lacquer acid is suspected to be the allergen. It is pointed out in *The Orthodox Manual of Wai Ke* that, "The response to lacquer varies greatly from person to person. Some people are (easily) susceptible and others remain unaffected (under the same circumstances)".

Diagnosis: Affected areas are mostly the exposed parts of the body, especially the face, neck, areas adjacent to the wrist, the back of the hand, and fingers. It may take the form of either papular erythema, vesicles, or even large-sized vesicles accompanied by ulcerations and suppuration. If it affects the face, the eyelids may be so puffy that the eyes can hardly open. In severe cases there may also be aversion to cold, fever, headache, and constipation or even mental confusion and insomnia.

Treatment

Internal Medication:

Hua Ban Jie Du Tang (35) or *Sheng Di Yin Hua Tang* (13) can be used to cool the blood, clear the heat, and resolve toxins.

External Therapies:

1) Make a cold compress made from the juice of 30 grams each of Herba Cum Radice Taraxaci Mongolici (*Pu Gong Ying*), Radix Sanguisorbae (*Di Yu*), and raw Radix Glycyrrhizae (*Sheng Gan Cao*).

2) Apply externally the juice from macerated fresh Folium Nelumbinis Nuciferae (*He Ye*) and fresh Herba Violae Yedoensis (*Zi Hua Di Ding*).

3) Mix *Qing Dai San* (20) into a paste with cold, boiled water and apply. Be sure enough water is used so that the area remains moist.

5. Dermatitis Medicamentosa
Yao Wi Xing Pi Yan

Pathogenesis and pathophysiology: This condition is due to an allergic response to certain chemicals. This type of skin rash involves the lungs since the lungs govern the superficial part of the body. When chemicals are dissolved in the stomach, they are distributed over (the body through) the blood vessels and ascend to the lungs. However, in the case of exfoliative dermatitis, chemical toxicity is also believed to be responsible above and beyond just an allergic reaction. Sulfa drugs, pain killers, antipyretics, antibiotics (including penicillin, sumycin, streptomycin), and sleeping pills (phenobarbital) may all cause allergic skin reactions.

Diagnosis: Some medicine causing the allergy has been taken. Typically, in such cases, there will be an incubation period. Skin reactions may occur from five to twenty days after such drugs are taken for the first time. However, in exfoliative dermatitis, the incubation period often exceeds twenty days. As for the morphology of the skin reaction, there can be great variation. There may be "ninth day" erythema (or fixed erythema), measle-like erythema, scarlatina-like erythema, urticaria-like erythema, multiform erythema, epidermolytic erythema with large vesicles, or exfoliative dermatitis.

Treatment

First stop using any suspected drugs.

Internal Medication:

Based on the principles of clearing heat, eliminating dampness, and resolving toxins, (decoct) Herba Cum Radice Taraxaci Mongolici (*Pu Gong Ying*) and Flos Lonicerae Japonicae (*Jin Yin Hua*), 15g @; Fructus Forsythiae Suspensae (*Lian Qiao*), Fructus Gardeniae Jasminoidis (*Shan Zhi Zi*), Radix Rubrus Paeoniae Lactiflorae (*Chi Shao*), Cortex Sclerotii Poriae Cocoris (*Fu Ling Pi*), Semen Plantaginis (*Che Qian Zi*), Rhizoma Alismatis (*Ze Xie*), and prepared Radix

21

Et Rhizoma Rhei (*Zhi Da Huang*), 10g @; and Radix Glycyrrhizae (*Gan Cao*), 3g. In case of constipation, use raw Radix Et Rhizoma Rhei (*Sheng Da Huang*) instead of prepared and add at the end. For those whose skin condition is scarlet colored, add Radix Rehmanniae (*Sheng Di*), 25g, and Cortex Radicis Moutan (*Dan Pi*), 10g. For severe pruritus, add Radix Sophorae Flavescentis (*Ku Shen*) and Cortex Radicis Dictamni (*Bai Xian Pi*), 10g @. For high fever, add Rhizoma Coptidis Chinensis (*Huang Lian*), Radix Scutellariae Baicalensis (*Huang Qin*), and Radix Scrophulariae Ningpoensis (*Xuan Shen*) and Tuber Ophiopogonis Japonicae (*Mai Dong*), 10g @, and fresh Herba Dendrobii (*Sheng Shi Hu*), 15g. If heat has entered the *ying* and blood phases, *Qing Ying Tang* (36) with modifications is advised to clear the *ying,* resolve toxins, and enrich yin so as to release heat.

External Therapies:

1) *San Huang Xi Ji* (28) is often employed externally to lesions restricted to a limited area, while *Qing Dai Gao* can be dusted over more extensive lesions. If a crust has formed or the affected area is dry, *Qing Dai Gao* can be used externally.

2) For moist exfoliative dermatitis it is preferable to apply *Qing Dai Gao* (20) as a lotion made with dilute, roasted sesame oil, 2-3 times per day. The area covered by this paste should be kept wet with sesame oil. As for scaling exfoliative dermatitis, a small amount of roasted sesame oil is likewise indispensable for protecting the skin. If there is a thick crust, use cotton swabs to gently anoint the area.

6. Eczema
She Zheng

Pathogenesis and pathophysiology: Eczema is called *jin yin chuang* (suppurative ulcerous lesion) in the classics. The six external evils are external causes and spleen dampness is its primary internal cause. Blood heat and wind heat are secondary causes. As an allergic dermatitis, the specific allergen (according to modern Western medicine) is hard to identify. (However,) it is believed that certain foods, intestinal parasites, infectious lesions, and spontaneous sensitivity or even cold (weather), wind, heat, sunlight, and certain plants can cause this condition. Eczema may also be related to the individual constitution and functional impairment of the nervous system.

Diagnosis

Acute Eczema: Acute eczema tends to appear abruptly and systematically on the interior aspects of the four extremities, such as at the cubital and popliteal fossae. It may also affect the face and neck, the dorsal aspect of the hands and feet, and the scrotum. Its manifestations are multiform: erythema, papules, watery blisters, pustules, suppurative ulcerations, and scabs. Two or three or even more of the above signs may present simultaneously. (However,) the border of the affected area *is always indistinct*. There may also be paroxysms of itching.

Chronic Eczema: Chronic eczema may either develop from acute eczema or it may develop by itself. It is characterized by rough, thickened skin, lichenification, desquamation, and pigment sedimentation *with a distinct border*. The patient often complains of sever itching. There may be frequent acute flare-ups on any part of the body; although the most commonly affected areas are the face, retroauricular region, the scrotum, and the shanks. Symptoms falling between acute and chronic forms are called subacute eczema.

Treatment

Internal Medication:

(In order) to clear heat and eliminate dampness in acute eczema a combination of *Bi Xie Shen Shi Tang* (8) and *Er Miao Wan* (37). These can be modified as follows: For upper body lesions, add Folium Mori Albi (*Sang Ye*), 10g, Flos Chrysanthemi Morifolii (*Ju*

23

Hua), 15g, and Periostracum Cicadae (*Chan Tui*), 3g, and delete Cortex Phellodendri (*Huang Bai*) and Sclerotium Poriae Cocoris (*Fu Ling*). For eczema over the abdominal region, add Rhizoma Coptidis Chinensis (*Huang Lian*) and Radix Scutellariae Baicalensis (*Huang Qin*), 10g @, and delete Cortex Phellodendri (*Huang Bai*). For eczema on the lower limbs, add Radix Achyranthis Bidentatae (*Niu Xi*) and Semen Plantaginis (*Che Qian Zi*), 10g @. And if there is constipation, add raw Radix Et Rhizoma Rhei (*Sheng Da Huang*), 10g after the decoction is well cooked.

Chronic eczema is treated by nourishing the blood, dispelling wind, and stopping itching. Either the combination of *Si Wu Tang* (38) with *Xiao Feng San* (3) with modifications or modified *Di Huang Yin* (10) may be used. For subacute eczema, treatment will depend upon the specific signs and symptoms. Some modification of acute and chronic treatments are often applied.

External Therapies

Acute Eczema

1) *San Huang Xi Ji* (26) is preferable for external use.

2) A cold compress can be made from a decoction of Radix Sophorae Flavescentis (*Ku Shen*) and Cortex Phellodendri (*Huang Bai*), 30g @, Cortex Radicis Dictamni (*Bai Xian Pi*) and Rhizoma Atractylodis (*Cang Zhu*), 15g @, and raw Radix Glycyrrhizae (*Sheng Gan Cao*), 30g.

Chronic Eczema

1) *Qing Dai Gao* (20) may be used externally.

2) Wash the affected area with a warm decoction of Radix Sophorae Flavescentis (*Ku Shen*) and Folium Mori Albi (*Sang Ye*), 30g @, Fructus Cnidii Monnieri (*She Chuang Zi*), Cortex Phellodendri (*Huang Bai*), and

Radix Sophorae Subprostratae (*Shan Dou Gen*), 15g @.

3) Fumigation therapy can be applied once or twice per day.

Subacute cases are treated by modulating the above protocols.

7. Aural Eczema
Er Bu Shi Zheng

Pathogenesis and Pathophysiology: The classic name for this pathology is *xuan er chuang* (lesion spiralling the ear) or eczema behind the ear. Its causes are typically similar to *jin yin chuang* above. However, this condition may also involve damp heat of the liver and gallbladder.

Diagnosis: Extensive erythema may appear in the creases behind the ears or spread over the retroauricular area. Exfoliation, suppurative ulceration, and scabs may recur and cause the lymph nodes behind the ear to swell. This condition is most commonly found in infants.

Treatment

Internal Medication:

Treatment of this condition should be aimed at clearing and eliminating dampness and heat from the liver and gallbladder. For this purpose, *Long Dan Xie Gan Tang* (39) is indicated.

External Therapies:

1) Finely pulverize raw Radix Et Rhizoma Rhei (*Sheng Da Huang*), 240g, Rhizoma Atractylodis (*Cang Zhu*), 40g, Realgar (*Xiong Huang*) and Alum (*Ku Fan*), 30g @, and Cortex Phellodendri (*Huang Bai*) 90g. Mix with roasted sesame oil before applying to affected area.

2) Use *Pi Zhi Gao* (40) externally.

3) In *Personal Experience in Wai Ke* it says "*Lian Ge San* is especial-
ly designed to treat infantile eczema." (This prescription consists of)
Rhizoma Coptidis Chinensis (*Huang Lian*) and pulverized Gecko (*Ge
Fen*), 3g @, Alum (*Ku Fan*), 1.5g, Realgar (*Xiong Huang*), Os
Sepiae Seù Sepiellae (*Hai Piao Xiao*), and Cortex Phellodendri
(*Huang Bai*), 3g @, Borneolum Syntheticum (*Bing Pian*), 0.3g, and
Indigo Naturalis (*Qing Dai*), 3g. Grind into a fine powder and mix
with roasted sesame oil before applying externally.

8. Cracked Nipple Complicated by Eczema
Ru Tou Jun Lie Xing Shi Zheng

Pathogenesis and pathophysiology: This is also called *ru tou feng* (nipple
wind) in the classics. Failure to discharge liver fire and accumulation
of damp heat in the *yang ming* are the causes. It is also believed that
the baby's suckling and the stimulation of their saliva are also factors.
In *Qian Yi-zhai's Case Histories in Wai Ke* written by Gao Jin-ting,
it is pointed out that, "Nipple wind itches when (the *yang ming*) are
obstructed and it is painful when being sucked."

Diagnosis: At its onset, the nipple feels itchy. Epidermal exfoliation,
cracked nipple, suppuration, and scabbing are common. Most cases
are found in breast-feeding primiparae.

Treatment

1) Mix finely powdered Radix Angelicae (*Bai Zhi*) with warm breast
milk and apply to the nipple.

2) *Qing Dai Gao* (20) can be applied externally.

3) According to *Emergency Prescriptions*, "Flos Caryophylli (*Ding
Xiang*) can be smashed and applied externally."

9. Eczema Around the Hip
Tun Bu Shi Zheng

Pathogenesis and pathophysiology: This condition is called *zuo ban chuang* (sitting board skin disease) in the classics. It is similar to *jin yin chuang* in origin. However, in it damp heat and toxins are predominant. According to its description in *Revealing the Mystery of Wai Ke*, "This condition results from long term accumulation of damp heat and damp toxins in the spleen channel which eventually gives rise to the most painful itching around the hip."

Diagnosis: Papules, desquamation, and lichenification may appear around the hip with hypertrophic skin. Itching may come and go. When scratched, the affected area produces fluid.

Treatment

Internal Medication:

Same as the treatment for *jin yin chuang*.

External Therapies

1) Grind into a fine powder Semen Phaseoli Munginis (*Lu Dou*), 30g, Cortex Phellodendri (*Huang Bai*), 10g, mercurous chloride Calomelas 6g, and Talcum (*Hua Shi*), 15g. Mix with roasted sesame oil and apply externally.

2) Wash or use a hip bath with *Ku Shen Tang* (30).

3) Use *Pi Zhi Gao* (40) externally.

4) According to *The Golden Mirror of Ancestral Medicine*, "Washing with hot water made from Flos Daphnis Genkwae (*Yuan Hua*), Fructus Zanthoxyli Bungeani (*Chuan Jiao*), and Cortex Phellodendri

(*Huang Bai*) can relieve the initial symptoms instantly (if applied in time)."

10. Scrotal Eczema
Yin Nang She Zheng

Pathogenesis and pathophysiology: Called *shen nang feng* (kidney sack wind) or *xiu qiu feng* (embroidered bell wind) in the ancient classics, its pathogenic factors are similar to that of *jin yin chuang* (in general) but with damp heat in the liver channel predominant. It is recorded in *The Golden Mirror of Ancestral Medicine* that, "Called *xiu qiu feng*, this condition is marked by itching of the scrotum. Accumulation of damp heat in the liver channel and the invasion of the surface by external wind evil are responsible."

Diagnosis: This condition is of two kinds: 1) dry and 2) ulcerous. Both forms are extremely tenacious in nature. They are characterized by severe itching, especially at night.

In the first type, the affected areas are often found covered with tiny scaling or grayish brown scabs. Hypertrophy of the skin, coarseness, and infiltrative lesions are prominent and may be accompanied by lichenification and scratching. In the second type, the affected area appears pink and dark red with ulcerated surface and fluid discharge which often stains the underwear. In some cases, ulceration may continue beneath the scab and secondary infection may also be present.

Treatment

Internal Medication:

For the first type, treatment should be based on cooling the blood, dispelling wind, and stopping itching. The indicated formula consists of Flos Chrysanthemi Morifolii (*Ju Hua*), 10g, Cortex Radicis Moutan (*Dan Pi*), 5g, Caulis Lonicerae Japonicae (*Ren Dong Teng*),

15g, Radix Rubrus Paeoniae Lactiflorae (*Chi Shao*), 5g, Fructus Kochiae (*Di Fu Zi*), 10g, and *Liu Yi San* (Talcum [*Hua Shi*] and Radix Glycyrrhizae [*Gan Cao*]), 10g. For the ulcerous type, treatment should focus on fortifying the spleen, eliminating dampness, and clearing heat for which one should take Radix Codonopsis Pilosulae (*Dang Shen*), Rhizoma Atractylodis Macrocephalae (*Bai Zhu*), Sclerotium Poriae Cocoris (*Fu Ling*), Rhizoma Alismatis (*Ze Xie*), Sclerotium Polypori Umbellati (*Zhu Ling*), Herba Pyrrosiae (*Shi Wei*), Fructus Chaenomelis Lagenariae (*Mu Gua*), Radix Astragali Membranacei (*Huang Qi*), and raw Semen Coicis Lachryma-jobi (*Sheng Yi Ren*), 15g @, and Semen Plantaginis (*Che Qian Zi*) and Radix Glycyrrhizae (*Gan Cao*), 5g @.

External Therapies:

For the dry type:

2) Wash with the water of Fructus Cnidii Monnieri (*She Chuang Zi*) and Cortex Phellodendri (*Huang Bai*), 30g @.

For the ulcerous type:

1) Smash several Fructus Canarii (*Gan Lan*), boil over a mild fire, and allow the juice to sit for 30 minutes before removing the dregs. Make a cold compress with this juice.

2) Make a cold compress with a decoction of Fructus Cnidii Monnieri (*She Chuang Zi*), Radix Glycyrrhizae (*Gan Cao*), and Cortex Phellodendri (*Huang Bai*), 30g @.

11. Eczema of the Hand
Shou Bu Shi Zheng

Pathogenesis and pathophysiology: This condition is called *guo chuang* (blisterous lesion) in the classics. Its causative factors (in general) are similar to *jin yin chuang* but in this case wind and damp pathogens predominate. *Personal Experience in Wai Ke* states, "Hand eczema is likely to develop between the fingers and the palm. The shape of the lesions often looks like Fructus Corni Officinalis (*Shan Zhu Yu*). This condition is not only characterized by yellowish and whitish pustules which discharge yellowish pus if perforated, but also by unpredictable bouts of itching. This condition results from the invasion of the surface of the body by wind and damp evils."

Diagnosis: Papules, vesicles, pustules, and ulceration are typically present and may attack repeatedly and symmetrically. Mycosis tests are negative.

Treatment

Internal Medication:

Same as for the treatment of *jin yin chuang*.

External Therapies:

1) Make a cold compress with a decoction of Cortex Phellodendri (*Huang Bai*), Radix Glycyrrhizae (*Gan Cao*), and Radix Sanguisorbae (*Di Yu*), 30g @.

2) Grind Colophonium (*Song Xiang*), 100g, Aerugo (*Tong Lu*), 240g, prepared Gypsum Fibrosum (*Shi Gao*), 100g, and prepared Alum (*Ku Fan*), 180g, into a fine powder and mix with sesame oil before use.

12. Periumbilical Eczema
Qi Bu Shi Zheng

Pathogenesis and pathophysiology: The classic name for this condition is *ji chuang* (umbilical lesion). It is related to irritation due to bathing and diapers. Qi Kun points out in *A Compendium of Wai Ke* (1665) that, "Eczema around the navel results from injury of the umbilicus by water dampness."

Diagnosis: Mostly this condition happens to infants. The umbilicus is typically wet due to fluid discharge. The area around the navel usually appears red. There is ulceration, small papules, and itching. If it is complicated with infection, the affected area is productive of purulent pus.

Treatment

External Therapy

1) *Sheng Ji San, i.e.*, grind Alum (*Ku Fan*) and prepared Os Draconis (*Duan long Gu*), 6g @ and Secretio Moschi Moschiferi (*She Xiang*), 0.3g, into a fine powder and dust this over the navel. If complicated by infection, a hot compress is recommended made from a decoction of Radix Glycyrrhizae (*Gan Cao*) and Cortex Phellodendri (*Huang Bai*), 30g @.

13. Infantile Eczema
Ying Er She Zheng

Pathogenesis and pathophysiology: This is called *tai lian chuang* (fetal astringency lesion) in the classics and its pathogenesis is similar to *jin yin chuang*. However, this condition is mainly due to the body's intolerance (to fetal toxins) and the accumulation of wind, dampness, and heat in the skin.

Diagnosis: This condition may appear in babies as young as one month old or in one to two year old infants. The superficial lesions manifest as tiny papules, vesicles, the discharge of pus, and scabs. They tend to appear symmetrically on the cheeks or spread to the area beneath the chin and neck. In severe cases, the shoulders, arms, lower limbs, and hip areas may also be affected.

However, even if lesions spread extensively, the center of the face, (e.g.) the area around the mouth and nose, is not involved. This condition tends to attack babies fed with nutritious food, who look chubby but not sturdy and in whom legs appear disproportionately (thin as compared) to their chubby cheeks.

Treatment

Internal Medication:

In order to clear heat, dispel wind, and eliminate dampness, *Xiao Feng Dao Che Tang* is preferred. (It is composed of) Radix Rehmanniae (*Sheng Di*) and Sclerotium Rubrum Poriae Cocoris (*Chi Fu Ling*), 9g @, Fructus Arctii (*Niu Bang Zi*), Cortex Radicis Dictamni (*Bai Xian Pi*), Flos Lonicerae Japonicae (*Jin Yin Hua*), Herba Menthae (*Bo He*), and Caulis Akebiae Mutong (*Mu Tong*), 6g @, and Rhizoma Coptidis Chinensis (*Huang Lian*), Radix Glycyrrhizae (*Gan Cao*), and Medulla Junci (*Deng Xin Cao*), 2g @. Decoct with water and take. Rhizoma Atractylodis (*Cang Zhu*) and Talcum (*Hua Shi*), 6g @, may be added in case of profuse fluid discharge. Add Radix Ledebouriellae Sesloidis (*Fang Feng*), 5g, for severe itching. Add Radix Scutellariae Baicalensis (*Huang Qin*), 3g, for mild infections and Flos Chrysanthemi Morifolii (*Ju Hua*), 6g, for hot, reddish skin.

External Therapies: For those with fluid discharge and ulceration, cold compresses are advised made from Cortex Phellodendri (*Huang Bai*) and Radix Glycyrrhizae (*Gan Cao*), 30g @, while powdered Rhizoma Coptidis Chinensis (*Huang Lian*), 20g, mixed with roasted sesame oil (*Xiang You*), 6g, can be used if fluid discharge is scanty or absent. (Another alternative is) to use *Qing Dai San* (20) after mixing it with roasted sesame oil. It is suggested in *The Golden Mirror of Ancestral Medicine* that, "*Run Ji Gao* (22) is indicated for dry (infantile eczema); while in cases with fluid discharge, dust (the affected area) with a mixture of equal parts Talcum (*Hua Shi*) and powdered sprouts of Radix Phellodendri (*Huang Bai Tou Wei*)."

Two

Urticarias

1. Urticaria
Qian Ma Zheng

Pathogenesis and pathophysiology: Urticaria is called *pei lei* (budding) in the classics. This condition is often caused either by dampness existing in the surface of the body complicated by wind heat or wind cold or by damp heat accumulating in the intestines and the stomach and dysfunction of the *chong* and *ren* due to irregularity of the organism. (According to modern Western medicine,) causative factors may include allergens such as fish, shrimp, and crab; certain medications; insect bites; contact with certain plants; internal infections; intestinal parasites; and functional impairment of the digestive tract. Exposure to cold, heat, wind, and light and emotional factors may also be causative agents. Local edema (*i.e.*) the wheal, is due to any of these causative factors causing the histocytes in the skin to release histoammonium thus causing dilation of the tiny blood vessels and increased permeability of the walls of the blood vessels.

Diagnosis: Wheals may appear suddenly and may also disappear within several hours. Typically they recur in groups incessantly. The patient may have outbreaks of hives from once to several times per day. (In acute cases), no new wheals will usually appear after the first week. In chronic cases, urticaria may attack the patient repeatedly and last from weeks to years. The lesions take the form of reddish or whitish bumps of various sizes. In some cases there may be accompanying diarrhea followed by pain. The skin scratch test typically is positive and there is often an elevated acidophil leukocyte count.

Treatment

Internal Medication:

The suggested treatment plan for acute urticaria is to promote diaphoresis, dispel wind, and clear heat in order to eliminate dampness by administering modified *Xiao Feng Sen* (3). For chronic urticaria, one should consolidate the surface and dispel wind. *Yu Ping Feng San* (2) is often used as the core prescription with additional ingredients.

External Therapies:

The external treatments of both acute and chronic urticaria are quite similar.

1) Acupuncture: *He Gu* (LI 4), *Qu Chi* (LI 11), *Xue Hai* (Sp 10), *Zu Zan Li* (St 36), *San Yin Jiao* (Sp 6), and *Yang Ling Quan* (GB 34) can be needled to stop itching.

2) Wash externally with the juice of Folium Perillae Frutescentis (*Zi Su Ye*), 120g.

3) Apply externally a tincture made from Radix Stemonae (*Bai Bu*), 30g., and rice wine (*Huang Jiu*), 60g., which has steeped for one week.

2. Papular Urticaria
Qiu Zhen Xing Qian Ma Zheng

Pathogenesis and pathophysiology: Also known as *xi pi feng zheng* (delicate skin rash), this condition is primarily an allergic reaction of the skin to insects, such as fleas, bedbugs, ticks, mites, and mosquitos. Pathogenic wind and heat are believed to be involved.

Diagnosis: This condition is commonly found in infants and during the summer and fall. The body trunk and the proximal areas of the extremities are the most likely sites. The basic lesion is a puffy, red papule similar in shape to a shuttle and the size of a popped corn. At the center of the papule is a watery blister the size of a pinhead. There is often intolerable itching leading to secondary infection after scratching. Although the lesion may fade within one to two weeks, pigment sedimentation may not later be relieved. This condition may come and go cyclically afterwards as well.

Treatment

Internal Medication:

In order to dispel wind and clear heat so as to remove the pathogenic factors, use Radix Ledebouriellae Sesloidis (*Fang Feng*), 6g, Radix Lithospermi Seu Arnebiae (*Hong Tiao Zi Cao*), 10g, Radix Rehmanniae (*Sheng Di*), and Folium Istatidis (*Da Qing Ye*), 15g @, and Herba Spirodelae Seu Lemnae (*Fu Ping*) and carbonized Fructus Crataegi (*Shan Zha*), 10g @.

External Therapies: *Zhi Yang Ding* (25) or a 25% solution of *Bai Bu Ding* (Stemona tincture) are often used externally.

Three _____

Suppurative Dermatitis

1. Pustulosis (Impetigo)
Nong Bao Chuang

Pathogenesis and pathophysiology: Pustulosis is called both *huang shui chuang* (yellow water lesion) and *nong cao chuang* (pus nest lesion) in the classics. It results from the complicated condition of heat in the lung channel and dampness in the spleen channel. (According to modern Western medicine,) it is an acute, suppurative skin disease caused by staphylococcus or streptococcus It says in *The Orthodox Manual of Wai Ke*, "*Huang shui chuang* tends to appear in the form of yellowish blisters around the face, head, and ear lobes. (It is characterized by) copious discharge of serous fluid and intolerable itching." While in *The Golden Mirror of Ancestral Medicine* it says, "Impetigo may appear wherever the dribbling yellow fluid touches." These two quotations indicate that this condition may spread all over the body.

Diagnosis: Mostly this condition occurs in the summer and fall. The majority of patients are children who have been exposed to or come in contact with pruritic dermatitis, such as miliaria and eczema. Exposed portions of the body, such as the face and extremities, are the most likely to be attacked. The basic lesions are either clusters of pustulae the size of soy beans or larger or suppurative blisters transformed from watery areas. These are surrounded by an inflammatory areola. The walls of the blisters are so thin that they are perforated easily, thus presenting an ulcerous surface. Yellowish scabs may form when dry and no scars are left upon recovery. The degree of itchiness is variable. Usually the adjacent lymph nodes will be enlarged. If the pustulae have spread widely there may be aversion to cold, fever, and other systemic symptoms. In a certain number of cases, this condition may lead to nephritis as a secondary infection.

Treatment

External Therapies:

1) Apply *Qing Dai San* (20) externally after being mixing with roasted sesame oil (*Xiang You*).

2) Mix pulverized Radix Lithospermi Seu Arnebiae (*Zi Cao*) and Rhizoma Coptidis Chinensis (*Huang Lian*), 30g @, with roasted sesame oil (*Xiang You*) and apply externally to the affected area.

3) Wash with the juice of Radix Sanguisorbae (*Di Yu*) and Cortex Phellodendri (*Huang Bai*), 60g @.

2. Furunculosis (Boils)
Jie Zhong

Pathogenesis and pathophysiology: These are called *shu jie* (summer eruption) in the classics and are believed to be caused by invasion of pathogenic summerheat. They often present as the acute, suppurative infection of the hair follicles or the connective tissue of the hair follicles.

Diagnosis: This condition is apt to occur around the head, face, neck, and hip. The boils may take the form of small, hard nodes at the onset and localized redness of skin, swelling, heat, and pain may all be present. Later on the nodes become soft and a whitish yellowish, suppurating pin-head sized lesion may appear at the top of the boil. Recovery will not occur until the boil is perforated and the pus discharged. Boils often leave scars after recovery. The adjacent lymph nodes are often found to be enlarged. In severe cases, systemic symptoms such as fever, are also present.

Treatment

Internal Medication:

In order to clear summerheat and resolve toxins one can prescribe:

1) *Qing Shu Tang* (7);

2) A decoction of Flos Lonicerae Japonicae (*Jin Yin Hua*) and white Flos Chrysanthemi Morifolii (*Bai Ju Hua*), 30g @, plus Radix Glycyrrhizae (*Gan Cao*), 15g

3) Or modified *Wu Wei Xiao Du Yin* (12).

External Therapies:

1) Apply smashed, fresh Herba Portulacae (*Ma Chi Xian*) externally.

2) Use externally dilute *Si Huang San* (19).

3) Use either *Qian Chui Gao* (16) or *Tai Yi Gao* (17).

3. Folliculitis
Mao Nong Yan

Pathogenesis and pathophysiology: Being a mild form of suppurative infection of the hair follicles, the pathogenesis of this condition is similar to that of boils. (According to modern Western medicine,) either staphylococcus or streptococcus are responsible.

Diagnosis: This condition may spread as far as the scalp, neck, chest, back, hip, or pudenda. It often takes the form of follicular papules at first with an inflammatory areola surrounding the adjacent area. The

39

tips of the papules may become purulent quite quickly and produce pus within just a few days. They will heal gradually after the pus has been evacuated and no scars will be left.

Treatment

In most cases, it is not necessary to take medicine. (However,) external application of *San Huang Xi Ji* (28) as a lotion or *Si Huang San* (19) diluted with water (are helpful).

4. Sycosis Barbae
Xu Chuang

Pathogenesis and pathophysiology: Called *yang hu chuang* (goat's beard lesion) or *yian wuo chuang* (swallow's nest lesion) in the classics, the pathogenesis of this condition is similar to that of boils and is also caused by suppurative staphylococcus. *Personal Experience in Wai Ke* states, "*Yian wuo chuang* develops on the chin. Hence the name goat's beard lesion. At its onset, its size can vary from as small as millet to as big as a bean. It may expand to wherever the yellowish fluid reaches after perforation. Damp heat of the spleen and stomach is always found to be responsible."

Diagnosis: This condition appears in the area of the beard and especially on the upper lip and the chin. The lesions often take the form of pustules or inflammatory papules with a hair at the center. Itching, burning, or pain are often felt.

Treatment

Internal Medication:

Use the same prescription as for the treatment of boils.

External Therapies:

1) *Pi Zhi Gao* (40) may be used as a lotion

2) According to *Personal Experience in Wai Ke*, "This condition can be relieved by applying *Bi Yu San* as a lotion." This is composed of equal parts powdered raw Cortex Phellodendri (*Huang Bai*) and calcined flesh of Fructus Zizyphus Jujubae (*Da Zao*) mixed with roasted sesame oil (*Xiang You*).

5. Erysipelas
Dan Du

Pathogenesis and pathophysiology: Being a localized, acute infection of the skin and mucous membranes, erysipelas is often due to invasion of pathogenic wind and fire. (However, according to modern Western medicine) streptococcus is responsible. Infection of a minor skin wound is often the precipitating factor. *A Compendium of Wai Ke* states, "So-called erysipelas is a skin condition which appears as if it were painted red... It often appears bright red and dry. In this case, both fever and pain are present due to liver and heart fire."

Diagnosis: Erysipelas is characterized by sudden onset. The shanks and face are the most likely areas to be affected. Its most characteristic feature is massive, puffy edema that projects above the normal skin. Therefore, there is a distinct, obvious border between the normal skin and the affected area. Sometimes, watery blisters may also appear on the surface of the erythema. The affected area tends to expand swiftly and there may be localized inflammation and pain. The adjacent lymph nodes will be enlarged and systemic symptoms such as fever and rigor may also be present.

Treatment

Internal Medication:

If the skin condition is concentrated on the head or face, *Pu Ji Xiao Du Yin* (42) is suggested with modifications in order to dispel wind, clear heat, and resolve toxins. If the skin condition spreads along the flanks and lumbar region, the combination of *Hua Ban Jie Du Tang* (35) and *Chai Hu Qing Gan Tang* (43) with modifications is recommended in order to clear liver fire and eliminate damp heat. If the lesions appear on the lower limbs, it is preferable to regulate the *ying* phase, eliminate dampness, clear heat, and resolve toxins by administering both *Bi Xie Sheng Shi Tang* (8) and *Wu Sheng Tang* (44) with modifications.

External Therapies: Either *Yu Lu San* (26), *Jin Huang San* (18), or *Si Huang San* (19) can be mixed as powders with cold, boiled water and applied to the affected area.

6. Suboccipital Indurative Folliculitis
Zheng Gu Xia Ying Jie Xing Mao Nang Yan

Pathogenesis and pathophysiology: This condition is called *fa ji chuang,* (hairline lesion). Stagnant damp heat and fire toxins are the internal causes and the invasion of pathogenic wind is the external cause. It is a suppurative skin disease around the hairline of the suboccipital region caused (according to modern Western medicine) by a combination of infection by *Micrococcus pyogenes* and the individual's predisposition to form keloids. In *The Golden Mirror of Ancestral Medicine* it states, "This condition develops over the hairline of the back of the neck like a grain of corn, the tip of which looks whitish with a reddish base. It feels hard. It can also be very painful or itch as if being pricked or burnt. It produces profuse serous fluid upon perforation. (There are) also victims (whose condition) originates form internal causes, such as the accumulation of damp heat complicated by pathogenic wind."

Diagnosis: This condition arises and is localized between the occipital bone and the posterior hairline. It may manifest as pin-head shaped follicular papules and may spread extensively at its onset. Consequent degeneration may occur, such as clusters of irregularly shaped indurations girdling and paralleling the hairline. These feel hard on palpation and emit a purulent fluid when pressed. Quite often these hard spots are found to have several hairs growing from one spot. This condition is known for its protracted course.

Treatment

Internal Medication:

In order to clear heat and resolve toxins, *San Huang Wan* is suggested which is composed of Rhizoma Coptidis Chinensis (*Huang Lian*), Radix Scutellariae Baicalensis (*Huang Qin*), and Radix Et Rhizoma Rhei (*Da Huang*), 100g @. These should be ground into a fine powder and made into pills with honey the size of Chinese parasol tree seeds. Take 30 pills once per day.

External Therapies:

Hu Po Gao (is recommended) which is composed of starch, 30g, Crinis Carbonisatus (*Xue Yu Tan*), 24g, mercurous chloride Calomelas, 12g, Cinnabaris (*Zhu Sha*), 21g, Fructus Zanthoxyli Bungeani (*Chuan Jiao*), 3g, Cera Flava (*Huang La*), 120g, Succinum (*Hu Po*), 2g, roasted sesame oil (*Xiang You*), 360g. Fry the Crinis Carbonisatus and Fructus Zanthoxyli Bungeani in the sesame oil until they are burnt and then remove the dregs. Melt the Cera Flava and then mix it with the starch, Cinnabaris, mercurous chloride Calomelas, and Succinum and mix all the above together to form a paste for external application.

7. Suppurative, Perforating Perifolliculitis
Nong Zhong Chuang Chu Xing Tou Bu Mao Nang Zhou Wei Yan

Pathogenesis and pathophysiology: This condition is called *lou gu jie* (mole cricket lesion) in the medical classics and is believed to be related to a vacuous constitution. (According to modern Western medicine,) it is due to bacterial infection and irritation of the skin by foreign bodies. *The Golden Mirror of Ancestral Medicine* states, "This condition, nicknamed *he nao*, often develops on the heads of children. Before perforation, the shape of the lesion resembles the head of a mole cricket. This condition becomes (so ulcerous) after perforation that it looks like a nest of mole crickets (with connecting underground pathways). One of the causes is *tai du* (*i.e.*, fetal toxins). In spite of the fact that the swelling is not so remarkable, it is a deep-rooted condition and the base of the wound will not turn tender even when there is perforation and discharge of pus. It often relapses even after scales have formed."

Diagnosis: As a deep-rooted folliculitis, this condition arises in the hair. Later it develops into perifolliculitis which continues to aggravate until there is a purulent, connective network of lesions. If the surface of the skin is pressed, pus will come out of most of the hair pores in the affected area. This is an ethmoid purulent discharge. The hairs in the diseased area fall and will not grow back again. This condition is characterized by its obstinate nature and prolonged course as well as by its tendency to recur. The atrophic scars never fade after recovery.

Treatment

Internal Medication:

In order to fortify the spleen and eliminate dampness, administer *Jian Pi Sheng Shi Tang* (9).

External Therapies: (Drain the pus by) lancing through the suppurative pathways and leave no hiding places for the pus. *Lin Yao Gao* (45) can be applied after the wound has been washed with a decoction of Flos Chrysanthemi Indici (*Ye Ju Hua*) and has been allowed to dry.

8. Chronic Ulcers on the Shank
Man Xing Xia Tui Kuei Yang

Pathogenesis and pathophysiology: *Lian chuang* (shank ulcer) is the name of the condition in the classics. Caused by the accumulation of damp heat in the lower extremities and complicated by the obstructed circulation of *ying* and blood, it may accompany the presence of varicose veins. Causative factors include dirty skin, wounds, insect bites, eczema, standing for prolonged periods, etc. *Revealing the Mystery of Wai Ke* states, "Due to damp toxins, contusions, wounds, scratches, insect bites, and dog bite, it is lingering in nature."

Diagnosis: The skin lesion may be composed of a number of separate ulcerations which may be circular, oblong, or irregular in shape with either distinct or indented borders. The granulation tissue looks pale and is covered by (a layer) of fatty fibroid tissue. The lesions are productive of mucoid excreta. There may also be necrosis of the surface with adjacent areas feeling hard and tense. As a rule, the ulceration is shallow. However, in some cases, the muscular membrane may also be involved. The subjective symptoms include light pain or itching. There may also be paroxysms of severe pain if neuroma develop along the borders of the affected area. This condition is characterized by its protracted course. It takes months or even years to heal.

Treatment

Internal Medication:

In order to nourish the blood, regulate the *ying* phase, eliminate dampness, and remove obstruction from the channels, *Bei Xie Hua Du Tang* is indicated: Rhizoma Dioscoreae Hypoglaucae (*Bie Xie*) and

45

Fructus Chaenomelis Lagenariae (*Mu Gua*), 12g @, Radix Angelicae Sinensis (*Dang Gui*), Cortex Radicis Moutan (*Dan Pi*), Radix Achyranthis Bidentatae (*Niu Xi*), Radix Stephaniae Tetrandrae (*Fang Ji*), and Radix Gentianae Macrophyllae (*Qin Jiao*), 9g @, and Semen Coicis Lachryma-jobi (*Yi Ren*), 30g. Decoct with water and take.

External Therapies:

1) A medicated wash can be made from Radix Ligustici Wallachii (*Chuan Xiong*), Radix Angelicae (*Bai Zhi*), and Ootheca Mantidis (*Sang Piao Xiao*), 15g @.

2) Apply *Sheng Ji Gao* (21) externally.

9. Ulceration of the female external genitalia
Nu Yin Kuei Yang

Pathogenesis and pathophysiology: The literal name of this condition is *yin shi* (erosion of private parts). It is caused either by a lack of hygiene of the external genitalia which gives rise to invasion of parasites or by heat derived from stagnant dampness. Examination of the vaginal discharge reveals the presence of *Bacillus crassus* which is presumed (by modern Western medicine) to be related to this condition.

Diagnosis: This condition typically presents at the commissure, especially the interior aspect of the minor commissure. Clinically it is divided into two types:

1) The ulcerous or gangrenous variety is marked by fever and malaise. Although the ulcerous lesions are few in number, they cause deep pain.

2) The venereal variety is characterized by an absence of any systemic symptoms and by large numbers of ulcerous lesions with shallow and slight pain. These are accompanied by nodular erythema and oral ulceration which often recur.

Treatment

Internal Medication:

In order to clear heat and eliminate dampness, administer *Long Dan Xie Gan Tang* (39) supplemented by Rhizoma Coptidis Chinensis (*Huang Lian*), 10g. Decoct with water and take.

External Therapies:

1) According to *The Golden Mirror of Ancestral Medicine,* (use) *Ta Yang Tang:* Radix Sophorae Flavescentis (*Ku Shen*), Radix Euphorbiae Kansui (*Gan Sui*), Fructus Cnidii Monnieri (*She Chuang Zi*), tails of Radix Angelicae Sinensis (*Gui Wei*), and Radix Clematidis (*Wei Ling Xian*), 15g @, Fructus Carpesii Abrotanoidis (*He Shi*), 30g, and bile from a pig's gallbladder (*Zhu Dan Ye*).

2) Another formula also called *Ta Yang Tang* (is found in) *The Medical Mirror of Wai Ke*: Fructus Cnidii Monnieri (*She Chuang Zi*), 30g, Fructus Zanthoxyli Bungeani (*Chuan Jiao*), 15g, and Alumen (*Ming Fan*), 9g. A decoction of the above can be used to steam the affected area when hot and to wash the area when it cools down some.

3) *Sheng Ji Gao* (21) can be applied externally.

Four _____

Fungal & Yeast Infections

1. Yellow Tinea Capitis
Huang Xian Xing Tou Xian

Pathogenesis and pathophysiology: This condition is called *fei chuang* (obesity lesion) in the classics and it is caused by pathogenic wind toxins. (According to modern Western medicine,) it is due to infection by the *Favus* fungus.

Diagnosis: The lesion on the scalp is a kind of crisp and adhesive, crust-like scab of variable size. It may be yellowish, grayish, or brownish in color. These scabs may emit a bad odor like mouse urine. Inflammation of the lesion is common. The disease progresses slowly and laboratory cultivation reveals (the existence of) *Favus*.

Treatment

Internal Medication:

In order to nourish the blood, dispel wind, and resolve toxins, administer Radix Sophorae Flavescentis (*Ku Shen*), Radix Polygoni Multiflori (*He Shou Wu*), and Radix Clematidis (*Wei Ling Xian*), 9g @, Radix Glycyrrhizae (*Gan Cao*) and Periostracum Cicadae (*Chan Tui*), 3g @, and Radix Rehmanniae (*Sheng Di*), 30g. Decoct in water and take.

External Therapies:

1) Wash the head with medicated water made from fresh Cacumen Biotae Orientalis (*Ce Bai Ye*), 120g.

2) Take 1 Nidus Vespae (*Feng Fang*), Scolopendra (*Wu Gong*), 2 pcs., and some Alumen (*Ming Fan*). Put the Alumen in the Nidus Vespae and bake together with the Scolopendra until they turn dark brown. Grind into powder and mix with roasted sesame oil before applying externally.

3) Take garlic juice (*Da Suan Ye*) 30g, lanolin (*Yang Mao Zhi*) 35g, and a combination of vegetable oil (*Cai You*) and Cera Flava (*Huang La*,) 35g. Mix the vegetable oil, Cera Flava, and lanolin before adding the garlic juice. Stir vigorously to prepare for external use. After applying to the scalp, wearing a hat is advised to prevent scratching.

4) *Da Zao San,* first recorded in *Personal Experience in Wai Ke*, is composed of Fructus Gleditschiae Chinensis (*Da Zao Jia*) and prepared Plastrum Testudinis (*Gui Ban*), 9g @ and raw Rhizoma Atractylodis (*Cang Zhu*), 15g. These should be fried until dark and powdered. Mix with roasted sesame oil (*Xiang You*) before use.

2. White Tinea Capitis
Bai Xian Xing Tou Xian

Pathogenesis and pathophysiology: This condition is called *bai tou chuang* (white scabby head) in the classics. It results from the invasion of pathogenic wind toxins (according to Traditional Chinese Medicine) and from infection by ferruginous microsporia (according to modern Western medicine).

Diagnosis: The manifestations of this condition are circular plaques. The hairs over the affected area are broken and therefore indented two to four millimeters up from the scalp. Also, the hairs around the whitish border of the ring fall off easily. This condition progresses quickly for the first two to three months. It then becomes static and ceases to expand. Cultures indicate the presence of ferruginous microsporia.

Treatment

1) Use the same treatments as for yellow tinea capitis.

2) According to *Revealing the Mystery of Wai Ke*, "*Xu You Gao* effects a magical cure in the treatment of scabby head that has not been cured for years." The method for preparing *Xu You Gao* is as follows: Take some Semen Momordicae Cochinensis (*Mu Bei Zi*) and stir fry it in vegetable oil until it turns black. Remove the dregs and add a mixture of 3/4 mercuric chloride Calomelas and 1/4 powdered Alumen (*Ming Fan*). Make into a paste for use.

3. Tinea Corporis
Ti Xian

Pathogenesis and pathophysiology: This is referred to as *dao xian* (knife tinea) or *yuan xian* (circular tinea) in the classics. This condition results from the invasion of the surface of the body by damp heat pathogens (from the tcm point of view) and is caused by mycosal infection (from the modern Western medical point of view).

Diagnosis: Most sufferers of tinea corporis are adults. It tends to occur in the summer and gets better in the winter. It is called tinea corporis because every part of the body is susceptible to it, except for the head, hands, feet, hips, fingers, and toes. The lower abdomen and waist are the most likely areas to be stricken. It manifests as circular plaques of various sizes with a clear border which is demarcated by pinhead-sized papules, watery blisters, pustules, scabs, or scaling and desquamation which stand in relief. (It is also characterized by) the tendency to heal in the center and to expand (on the periphery) and is accompanied by a subjective sensation of itching.

Treatment

For most cases, decoctions (administered internally) are unnecessary.

External Therapies:

1) Grind some Semen Momordicae Cochinensis (*Mu Bei Zi*) with vinegar in a ceramic pot. Apply the medicated juice externally 3 times per day.

2) Apply a medicated tincture made from Cortex Pseudolaricis (*Tu Jing Pi*), flesh of Semen Hydnocarpi (*Da Feng Zi*), Cortex Radicis Dictamni (*Bai Xian Pi*), Fructus Kochiae (*Di Fu Zi*), Fructus Cnidii Monnieri (*She Chuang Zi*), and Radix Sophorae Flavescentis (*Ku Shen*), 30g @, Sulphur (*Liu Huang*) and Camphor (*Zhang Nao*), 15g @, and Alumen (*Ming Fan*), 120g. Soak in 2000 ml. of 50% alcohol for one week.

4. Tinea Cruris (Jock Itch)
Gu Xian

Pathogenesis and pathophysiology: Another name for this condition is *yin xian* (private parts tinea). It is due to the same causes as tinea corporis.

Diagnosis: As its name implies, this condition affects the internal aspects of the thigh, the perineum, and the buttocks. The majority of sufferers are adults in whom it is likely to recur in the summer and be relieved in the winter. The lesions themselves are similar to tinea corporis in appearance.

Treatment

In most cases, internal medication is unnecessary.

External Therapies:

1) Mix well two egg yolks, Acacia Catechu (*Er Cha*), 3g, and Borneolum Syntheticum (*Bing Pian*), 0.3g, and apply externally.

2) Tincture in 1500g of white vinegar for 20 days fresh, chopped Rhizoma Opuntiae (*Xian Ren Zhang*), 90g, chopped Fructus Strophanthi Divaricati (*Yang Jia Ai Guo*), 150g, chopped Herba Wikstroemiae Indicae (*Liao Ge Wang*), 45g. and chopped Herba Adenosmae Glutinosae (*Mao She Xiang*), 30g. Remove dregs and apply externally.

5. Tinea Palmaris
Shou Xian

Pathogenesis and pathophysiology: This condition is referred to as *e zhang feng* (goose palm wind) in the classics. Heat in the spleen and stomach and wind due to blood heat are the causative factors. (According to modern Western medicine,) it is due to fungal infection. *A Compendium of Wai Ke* states, "At the onset, goose palm wind presents as (a series of) purpurae with white dots. (As it evolves,) the skin turns dry and thick. (Consequently,) fissures or cracks are inevitable."

Diagnosis: Tinea palmaris tends to appear between the fingers and on the palms. It may crawl to the dorsal aspect of the hand. It is typically aggravated during the summer and improves somewhat in winter. (As far as its) morphology, it is usually classified into three categories. Although all three may be simultaneously present, one variety is usually more pronounced.

1) Blister type: The lesions take the form of deep blisters with severe itching. Secondary infections my arise after scratching or pricking with needles in an attempt to relieve the intolerable itching sensation.

2) Erosive type: Most of the lesions lie between the fingers and especially between the third and fourth fingers. The surface of the skin is pale as if immersed in water, while the deep layers of the skin are scarlet and ulcerous. There is severe itching accompanied by pain. Secondary infection is also very possible.

3) Squamous cornification type: Here there is cornification and scaling over the palm with a pink base. There may or may not be itching. During the winter, when the skin cracks, there is pain.

Treatment

Internal medication need not be administered in most cases. (However,) *Qu Feng Di Huang Wan* is indicated for the treatment of the squamous cornification type in order to nourish the blood, moisten dryness, and eliminate wind. (It is composed of) Radix Rehmanniae (*Sheng Di*) and Radix Coquitus Rehmanniae (*Shu Di*), 120g @, white Fructus Tribuli Terrestris (*Bai Ji Li*) and Radix Achyranthis Bidentatae (*Niu Xi*), 90g @, Rhizoma Anemarrhenae (*Zhi Mu*), Cortex Phellodendri (*Huang Bai*), and Fructus Lycii Chinensis (*Gou Qi Zi*), 60g @, and Semen Cuscutae (*Tu Si Zi*) and Radix Duhuo (*Du Huo*), 30g @. Grind into fine powder and make into pills with honey. Take 10g each time, 1—2 times per day.

External Therapies:

1) Blister type: Tincture Flos Caryophylli (*Ding Xiang*), 20g in 100 ml of 70% alcohol for 7 days.

2) Erosive type: Dust with equal parts powdered Cortex Phellodendri (*Huang Bai*) and Alumen (*Ming Fan*) or use a cold compress made from the medicated juice of Radix Sophorae Flavescentis (*Ku Shen*), Fructus Cnidii Monnieri (*She Chuang Zi*), Fructus Xanthii (*Cang Er Zi*), Herba Agastachis Seu Pogostemi (*Huo Xiang*), and Alumen (*Bai Fan*), 30g @. As soon as the symptoms improve, *i.e.* the wound produces less serous fluid, use the same treatment as for tinea cruris.

3) Squamous Cornification type: Simmer two pieces of Nidus Vespae (*Feng Fang*) in 500ml of white vinegar until the liquid is reduced by half. Cool, strain, and apply externally, or use the same tincture as for tinea corporis, or use fumigation instead (32).

4) *Ku Shen Tang* (30) can be used externally for all varieties of this condition.

5) According to *Revealing the Mystery of Wai Ke*, "The formula for goose palm wind consists of powdered Mirabilitum (*Po Xiao*) mixed with Tung oil (*Tong You*). Heat over fire before applying to the affected area. (It will bring about) a wonderful effect in just a couple of treatments."

6) According to *A Compendium of Wai Ke*, use *Er Fan San* (which is composed of) Alumen (*Ming Fan*) and Melanteritum (*Qing Fan*), 30g @, Acacia Catechu (*Er Cha*), 15g, and Cacumen Biotae Orientalis (*Ce Bai Ye*), 60g. Heat and wash.

6. Tinea Pedis
Zu Xian

Pathogenesis and pathophysiology: This condition is due to the downward percolation of damp heat from the spleen and stomach channels. (According to modern Western medicine,) it is caused by fungal infection. In the classics, the erosive type is called *chou tian luo* (stinking river snail), while the blister type is called *tian luo bao* (river snail blisters).

Diagnosis:

1) Blister type: This condition tends to occur around the arch of the foot or on both sides of the toes. It can be composed of concentrated or scattered little blisters. As these become perforated or absorbed, they may produce a certain amount of scaling. With an increase in the number of blisters, semicircular or irregular shaped plaques may fall off. Recurrence of this condition renders the skin rough and thick and cracks develop easily in winter. (Moreover,) itching is also present. Secondary infection may turn the blisters into pustules with a burning sensation.

2) Erosive type: This type tends to occur between the toes, especially between the third and fourth toes. The skin looks pale due to moisture and is productive of fluid. A red wound surface is exposed when the skin is taken off. There is itching, pain, and a particular malodor.

3) Squamous cornification type: This tends to occur between the toes, on the sides of the heels, and on the soles. The symptoms are excessive cornification, dryness, roughness, desquamation, and rhagas. This type of tinea often evolves from the water blister type.

Treatment

Internal medication is not indicated for most cases. However, if complicated (by other signs or symptoms), one should clear heat, resolve toxins, and eliminate dampness by using Rhizoma Atractylodis (*Cang Zhu*), Fructus Gardeniae Jasminoidis (*Zhi Zi*), Cortex Phellodendri (*Huang Bai*), Radix Achyranthis Bidentatae (*Niu Xi*), Rhizoma Dioscoreae Hypoglaucae (*Bi Xie*), and Radix Glycyrrhizae (*Gan Cao*), 10g @, Flos Lonicerae Japonicae (*Jin Yin Hua*) and Fructus Forsythiae Suspensae (*Lian Qiao*), 15g @, and raw Semen Coicis Lachryma-jobi (*Sheng Yi Ren*), 30g. Decoct in water and take.

External Therapies:

1) Water blister type: Dust with a mixture of *Liu Yi San,* 30g, and Alumen (*Ming Fan*), 60g. (*Liu Yi San* is composed of Talcum [*Hua Shi*], 180g, and Radix Glycyrrhizae [*Gan Cao*], 30g.) An alternative treatment is to use the same tincture as in tinea palmaris of the watery blister variety. (According to) *The Golden Mirror of Ancestral Medicine*, "River snail blisters should be washed hot with the medicated juice made from Radix Sophorae Flavescentis (*Ku Shen*), Rhizoma Acorii Graminei (*Shi Chang Pu*), and wild Herba Artemesiae Argyii (*Qing Ai*). Then rip off the blisters and apply a mixture of powdered Gypsum Fibrosum (*Shi Gao*) and Calomelas (*Qing Fen*)."

2) Erosive type: Dust a mixture of equal parts powdered Rhizoma Atractylodis (*Cang Zhu*) and Cortex Phellodendri (*Huang Bai*). Or,

use the same external treatment as for tinea palmaris. In *The Golden Mirror of Ancestral Medicine* it says, "Stinking river snail should be washed with Radix Glycyrrhizae (*Gan Cao*) and Semen Coicis Lachryma-jobi (*Yi Yi Ren*)."

3) Squamous cornification type: Grind into a fine powder and mix together with roasted sesame oil (*Xiang You*) Cortex Phellodendri (*Huang Bai*), Semen Arecae Catechu (*Bing Lang*), and Rhizoma Atractylodis (*Cang Zhu*), 10g @, and Borneolum Syntheticum (*Bing Pian*), 3g. An alternative therapy is to employ the same formula as for squamous cornification tinea palmaris.

4) *Ku Shen Tang* (30) is applicable to all varieties of this condition.

7. Tinea Unguium
Jia Xian

Pathogenesis and pathophysiology: This condition is also called *hui jia* (ashy nail) or *e zhua feng* (goose-claw wind). Its pathogenesis is similar to tinea palmaris. It is a fungal infection.

Diagnosis: The finger and toenails lose their normal shape and color. They lose their lustre, become fragile and may become either atrophic or hypertrophic. (In addition,) the finger or toenails are often found separated from the nail bed. In most cases, tinea unguium will not evolve into paronychia unless it becomes infected by moniliasis. However, this condition is often a precursor to tinea palmaris or tinea pedis. Culturing and other tests are positive for fungus.

Treatment

In most cases, internal medication is unnecessary.

External Therapies:

1) Immerse the diseased nail in white vinegar for 20-30 minutes once per day.

2) Scrape the diseased nail with a blunt knife or file the nail every 5-7 days. Afterwards, apply a tincture 3 times per day made from the following ingredients: Cortex Pseudolaricis (*Tu Jing Pi*), 18g, Mylabris (*Ban Mao*), 15g, and prepared Realgar (*Xiong Huang*), 12g. Tincture in 500ml of white vinegar for one week before applying.

3) Cut into small pieces and tincture Herba Agastachis Seu Pogostemi (*Huo Xiang*), 30g, and Rhizoma Polygonati (*Yu Zhu*), Radix Et Rhizoma Rhei (*Da Huang*), and Melanteritum (*Qing Fan*), 12g @ in 500ml of white vinegar. Strain out the vinegar after one week. The patient should immerse the diseased nail in this tincture for at least 30 minutes every day. The total immersion (*i.e.* the total course of treatment) should total more than 24 hours. During this time it is preferable not to wash the hands with alkaline soap. Scrape or file the nail before soaking.

4) Smash white Herba Impatientis Balsaminae (*Bai Feng Xian Hua*) and mix with a small amount of powdered Alumen (*Ming Fan*). Apply to the diseased nail and hold in place with a large bandage. Change this dressing daily for 30 days.

8. Tinea Versicolor
Hua Ban Xian

Pathogenesis and pathophysiology: Tinea versicolor is called *bai dian feng* (white skin wind) or *li yang feng* (pestilential, ulcerous wind) in the classics. Its folk name is *han ban* (sweating marks). Tinea versicolor results from the accumulation of pathogenic wind in the skin (according to TCM) and from infestation by the tinea versicolor fungus (according to modern Western medicine). *A Compendium of Wai Ke* says, "*Bai dian feng* or leukoderma is nicknamed *han ban*. It appears purplish because of blood stasis and white because of qi stagnation. Both are due to invasion of the surface by wind and dampness. It is painless even if scratched." Tinea versicolor yeast can be found by testing.

Treatment

For most cases, internal medication can be avoided.

External Therapies:

1) Grind Radix Duhuo (*Du Huo*), 30g, Borneolum Syntheticum (*Bing Pian*), 1g, and Lithargyum (*Mi Tuo Seng*) and Sulfur (*Liu Huang*), 15g @, into a powder and mix with rice wine for use.

2) Apply externally a tincture made from Radix Stemonae (*Bai Bu*), 60g, Borax (*Peng Sha*), 6g, and rice wine (*Huang Jiu*), 250ml. Tincture the first two ingredients in the rice wine for from three to four days before use.

3) Take Fructus Momordicae Charantiae (*Ku Gua*), 1 piece (about 60g) and *Xing Shi* (a processed mixture of Arsenolitum, Arsenopyritum, and Realgar) 0.6g. Cut an opening in the end of the Fructus Momordicae Charantiae and put in the powdered *Xing Shi*. Wrap the fruit in two layers of wet toilet paper and bake until cooked. Take off the paper and wrap with gauze. Rub the affected part with this or apply the fluid pressed from the fruit instead. One day before this treatment the patient is advised to take a hot bath with soap and water. Two or three consecutive treatments can cure this condition.

9. Stacked Tile Tinea
Die Wa Xian

Pathogenesis and pathophysiology: Another name for this disease is *quan xian* (circular tinea). It is believed to be caused by invasion of the skin by pathogenic damp heat. The pathogenic microorganism (according to modern Western medicine) is a fungi.

Diagnosis: The skin lesions appear as small, squamous chips, spirallic or concentric in shape. They are characterized by their distinct margins. Although this condition most often affects the four extremities, it may attack any part of the body and even the junctures of the skin and mucosal membranes. However, the palm is seldom and the hair follicles are never involved. Itching may be present during its long course of development regardless of season. This condition is recalcitrant to treatment. Mycosal culture reveals the presence of fungi.

Treatment

1) Treat with the same methods as for tinea corporis.

2) Grind Radix Euphorbiae Pallasii (*Lang Du*), 9g, and Alumen (*Ming Fan*), Sulphur (*Liu Huang*), and Mylabris (*Ban Mao*), 3g @, into fine powder and mix well with some raw pig's fat. Rub the affected area with the pig's fat wrapped in gauze.

3) Crush Rhizoma Bletillae (*Bai Ji*), Radix Stemonae (*Bai Bu*), Semen Arecae Catechu (*Bing Lang*), Realgar (*Xiong Huang*), and Radix Aconiti (*Chuan Wu*), 60g @, Scolopendra (*Wu Gong*) 20pcs., Cortex Pseudolaricis (*Tu Jing Pi*), 120g, Periostracum Cicadae (*Chan Tui*), and white Arsenicum (*Bai Pi*), 9g @, and Mylabris (*Ban Mao*), 7pcs. Place in a cloth bag and tincture for one month in 4000 ml of rice wine (*Huang Jiu*). Remove the dregs and apply the tincture externally.

10. Dermatophytids or "Id" Eruptions
Xian Jun Zheng

Pathogenesis and pathophysiology: This condition is caused by pathogenic heat due to external wind evil and complicated by internal dampness. (According to modern Western medicine) it is a kind of allergic response of the skin to active tineasis present in the body.

Diagnosis: Active tinea lesions may appear on the hands, feet, or head in multiple shapes. The most common sign is groups of little water blisters on both hands. There is the subjective symptom of itching. There may also be occasional fever.

Treatment

Internal Medication:

In order to expel wind, eliminate dampness, and clear heat, administer (a decoction made from) Rhizoma Smilacis Glabrae (*Tu Fu Ling*), Flos Lonicerae Japonicae (*Yin Hua*), dried Radix Rehmanniae (*Gan Di Huang*), and Talcum (*Hua Shi*), 30g @, Radix Rubrus Paeoniae

Lactiflorae (*Chi Shao*), Semen Plantaginis (*Che Qian Zi*), and Cortex Radicis Dictamni (*Bai Xian Pi*), 10g @, and Periostracum Cicadae (*Chan Tui*) and Radix Glycyrrhizae (*Gan Cao*), 3g @.

External Therapies:

1) Use *San Huang Xi Ji* (28) externally.

2) Wash the affected area with a decoction made from Radix Sophorae Flavescentis (*Ku Shen*), Fructus Cnidii Monnieri (*She Chuang Zi*), Fructus Xanthii (*Cang Er Zi*), and Alumen (*Ming Fan*), 30g @.

11. Oral Candidiasis (Thrush)
Kou Qiang Nian Mo Nien Zhu Jun Bin E Kou Chuang

Pathogenesis and pathophysiology: Thrush is called *e kou chuang* (goose mouth sore) in the classics and is caused by heat in the heart, spleen, and lung channels. (According to modern Western medicine,) *Candida albicans* is the yeast responsible. *Personal Experience in Wai Ke* states, "Goose mouth sore (is characterized by) white dots all over the mouth. The majority of sufferers are children. It is caused by wind heat of the spleen and lung channels."

Diagnosis: Creamy white patches or a curdy substance appear over the oral mucosa, tongue, and pharyngeal membranes. Quite often these patches can be easily wiped off. In some cases, there may be blisters followed by swelling of the surrounding areas due to local congestion. The mouth may also feel inflamed. Typically, the patient is an infant. (Hyper)salivation may be induced during breast feeding. Vomiting and diarrhea may also be found.

Treatment

Internal Medication:

Treatment should be based on the principles of clearing heat, resolving toxins, and eliminating dampness.

1) To clear heat and drain the spleen: Prepared Gypsum Fibrosum (*Shi*

Gao), 18g, Rhizoma Coptidis Chinensis (*Hang Lian*) and Fructus Gardeniae Jasminoidis (*Shan Zhi Zi*), 6g @, Radix Rehmanniae (*Sheng Di*), 15g, Cortex Phellodendri (*Huang Bai*), and Radix Rubrus Paeoniae Lactiflorae (*Chi Shao*), 9g @, and Medulla Junci (*Deng Xin Cao*), 3g.

2) Modified *Dao Chi San:* Radix Rehmanniae (*Sheng Di*) and Flos Lonicerae Japonicae (*Jin Yin Hua*), 15g @, Herba Lopthatheri Gracilis (*Dan Zhu Ye*) and Fructus Gardeniae Jasminoidis (*Zhi Zi*), 9g @, Radix Scutellariae Baicalensis (*Huang Qin*), Caulis Akebiae Mutong (*Mu Tong*) and Semen Plantaginis (*Che Qian Zi*), 6g @. Decoct with water and take.

3) From *A Supplement to the Medical Profession, Niu Jie Tang:* Fructus Arctii (*Niu Bang Zi*) and Radix Platycodi Grandiflori (*Jie Gen*), 9g @, Radix Puerariae Lobatae (*Ge Gen*) and Bulbus Fritillariae Thunbergii (*Zhe Bei Mu*) 6g @, and Radix Bupleuri (*Chai Hu*), Radix Glycyrrhizae (*Gan Ca*), Fructus Citri Seu Ponciri (*Zhi Ke*), and Herba Menthae (*Bo He*), 3g @.

External Therapies:

1) Alumen (*Ming Fan*), burnt into ash, and Cinnabaris (*Zhu Sha*), ground into powder while adding water, 8g @, and crystallized Niter (*Ya Xiao*), 16g. Mix the above powdered ingredients with water before applying to the tongue, the inside of the mouth, and the angles of the mouth.

2) *Bing Peng San:* Grind Borneolum Syntheticum (*Bing Pian*), 3g, Cinnabaris (*Zhu Sha*), 3.5g, and prepared Borax (*Peng Sha*) and purified sodium sulfate, 30g @, into fine powder and dust (the affected area).

3) *Liu Qing San*: Grind Indigo Naturalis (*Qing Dai*), 6g, Herba Menthae (*Bo He*), 15g, Acacia Catechu (*Er Cha*), 24g, and Rhizoma Coptidis Chinensis (*Huang Lian*), 12g, into fine powder and mix with Borneolum Syntheticum (*Bing Pian*), 3g. Dust (the affected area) with this mixture.

Five _____

Cutaneous Tuberculosis

1. Scrofular Cutaneous Tuberculosis
Lei Li Xing Pi Fu Jie He

Pathogenesis and pathophysiology: Called *lie li* (scrofula) in the classics, this condition results from poor health, insufficiency of qi and blood, and accumulation of phlegm and turbidity in the channels and connecting vessels. (According to modern Western medicine,) it is caused by the proliferation of tubercular bacilli from tubercular lesions of the bones and lymph nodes.

Diagnosis: Typically this condition appears on the sides of the neck, under the armpits, and in the inguinal grooves or over the upper chest in children. Hard, moveable nodulations may be noted at the outset. Later, these nodes grow and connect with the skin. They gradually turn red and eventually become soft and perforated or ulcerous or fistulous. The margins of the ulceration are often occult and bundle-like scars are often produced after recovery. Adjacent nodulations may follow the same course of development and may connect with each other. (In such cases) finally the scars may look like a girdle. Histological changes show tubercular granuloma.

Treatment

Internal Medication:

1) In order to consolidate the qi and nourish the blood, administer *Ba Zhen Tang*: Radix Coquitus Rehmanniae (*Shu Di*), 24g, Radix Codonopsis Pilosulae (*Dang Shen*), 15g, Sclerotium Poriae Cocoris

(*Fu Ling*), 12g, Rhizoma Atractylodis Macrocephalae (*Bai Zhu*), Radix Angelicae Sinensis (*Dang Gui*), and Radix Albus Paeoniae Lactiflorae (*Bai Shao*), 9g @, Radix Praeparatus Glycyrrhizae (*Zhi Gan Cao*) and Rhizoma Ligustici Wallachi (*Chuan Xiong*), 5g @. Decoct in water and take. This decoction is indicated for those whose body is vacuous *i.e.*, suffer from constitutional vacuity.

2) In order to transform phlegm and soften the hard, *Hai Zao Yu Hu Tang* is often administered: Herba Sargassi (*Hai Zao*) and Herba Zosterae Marinae (*Hai Dai*), 12g @, Fructus Forsythiae Suspensae (*Lian Qiao*), Thallus Algae (*Kun Bu*), Radix Angelicae Sinensis (*Dang Gui*), and Rhizoma Pinelliae Ternatae (*Ban Xia*), 9g @, Bulbus Fritillariae Cirrhosae (*Chuan Bei Mu*), 6g, Pericarpium Viridis Citri Reticulatae (*Qing Pi*), Pericarpium Citri Reticulate (*Chen Pi*), Radix Duhuo (*Du Huo*), Radix Ligustici Wallichii (*Chuan Xiong*), and Radix Glycyrrhizae (*Gan Cao*), 5g @. This decoction is indicated for those whose body is replete.

External Therapies:

1) For those with ulcerous conditions, use wet compresses with a 20% tincture of Radix Stemonae (*Bai Bu*).

2) Mix equal portions of powdered Realgar (*Xiong Huang*), Alumen (*Ming Fan*), and Alum (*Ku Fan*) with petroleum jelly and apply externally.

3) After crushing, calcine Rhizoma Amorphophalli Rivieri (*Ju Ruo*), 100g, with mild fire until its surface becomes ashen. Grind and refine this and then mix with Tung oil (*Tong You*), 200g, or Oleum Ricini Communis (*Bi Ma You*) into a paste for external application. Change the dressing once per day.

2. Erythema Induratum
Ying Hong Ban

Pathogenesis and pathophysiology: This condition is similar to what is called *shan lou* (fistula of the calf) in the classics. It results from qi stagnation and blood stasis due to exhaustion of the three yin and obstruction of phlegm and dampness. (According to modern Western medicine,) this is due to tubercular bacilli. *The Golden Mirror of Ancestral Medicine* states, "*Shan lou* looks like eczema at the beginning. It appears on the back of the calf with alternating itching and pain. (Once it becomes perforated,) it persistently produces a yellowish fluid because of deep-rooted ulceration. In cases complicated by pathogenic wind, there may be a cold appearance and cold limbs."

Diagnosis: Most patients are young women. This condition tends to occur on the back of the calf. The basic lesion is a subcutaneous nodulation which grows and connects with the skin and turns purple in color. The nodulation does not necessarily protrude but it feels solid with slight pain upon pressure. It may resolve itself spontaneously or it may become ripe and perforate. In that case, there will be deep ulceration, irregular in shape. Accompanying symptoms such as fistula may also be present and excrete caseous fluid, thin and light yellow in color. Scars may be produced after healing. There will be soreness and pain. The course of development is characteristically long and there is likelihood of relapse. Tubercular skin patch test will be positive and histological change shows tubercular granuloma, although a few cases may be non-specific.

Treatment

Internal Medication:

In order to nourish the blood, enrich yin, and strengthen the spleen, *Liu Wei Di Huang Wan* (46) may be prescribed to be taken with a light salt solution, 12g each time, 2 times per day.

External Therapies:

1) *Chong He San*: Prepared Cortex Radicis Kadsurae (*Zi Jing Pi*), 150g, Radix Duhuo (*Du Huo*), 90g, Radix Rubrus Paeoniae Lactiflorae (*Chi Shao*), 60g, Rhizoma Acori Graminei (*Shi Chang Pu*), 45g, and Radix Angelicae (*Bai Zhi*), 30g. Grind these into a fine powder and mix with scallion juice (*Cong Ye*) and rice wine (*Huang Jiu*) before applying to the unperforated condition.

2) *Hua Hu Sheng Ji San*: Raw Gummi Olibanum (*Sheng Ru Xiang*) and raw Myrrha (*Sheng Mo Yao*), 15g @, Os Sepiae Seu Sepiellae (*Wu Zei Gu*) and Realgar (*Xiong Huang*), 9g @, Borax (*Peng Sha*), 30g, and Borneolum Syntheticum (*Bing Pian*), 3g. This prescription is indicated for perforated conditions. Spread petroleum jelly on a piece of gauze and cover this with the above powdered herbs. Apply to the affected area. This dressing should be changed once per day.

Six _____

Dermatitis Due to Viral Infection

1. Common Warts (Verrucae vulgaris)
Xun Chuang You

Pathogenesis and pathophysiology: Warts are called *qian ri chuang* (thousand day sores) or *ci hou* (thorny condition) in the classics. They are due to lingering pathogenic wind in the skin due to blood dryness and liver vacuity. (According to modern Western medicine,) they are a species of viral vegetation.

Diagnosis: This condition tends to occur on the dorsal aspect of the hands and feet, on the fingers and toes, and around the borders of the nails. Warts commonly take the form of circular papules of normal skin color or they may be brownish yellow. The size of warts may vary from that of a pinhead to that of a soybean or even larger with a rough uneven surface. They are not accompanied by any other subjective symptoms. Tenderness may be present if the warts occur at the edge of the nails. This condition typically progresses slowly and may resolve itself spontaneously in some cases.

Treatment

1) Boil Herba Equiseti Hiemalis (*Mu Zei*) and Rhizoma Cyperi Rotundi (*Xiang Fu*), 30g @, in 1500 ml of water. Wash and rub slightly the affected area twice per day, thirty minutes each time.

2) Disinfect the local area with 75% alcohol and then introduce 1% procaine injection in order to achieve local anesthesia. Next apply direct moxibustion to the wart(s) with a moxa roll. After moxibustion,

scrape the base of the wart with a knife to (completely) eradicate it. The wound should be dressed with gauze after applying a 2% solution of gentian violet.

3) Smash a kernel of Fructus Bruceae Javanicae (*Ya Dan Zi*) until oil (is squeezed out and) apply this oil to the warts once every other day.

4) Rub (the affected area) once per day with either fresh or dried Endothelium Corneum Gigeraiae Galli (*Ji Nei Jin*) after it has been softened by immersion in water.

2. Flat Warts
Bian Ping You

Pathogenesis and pathophysiology: Another name for this condition is *bian hou* (flat condition). They are caused by pathogenic wind and hot toxins externally and by flaring of liver fire internally. (According to modern Western medicine,) these are also a kind of viral vegetation.

Diagnosis: Most victims (of flat warts) are youths. They tend to be found on the face, forearms, and dorsal aspect of the hand. Such warts book like flat papules. They are normal skin color or light brown and are hard in quality. Their size may vary from that of a grain of rice to that of a soybean. Their surface is smooth to the touch and shiny. In most cases, there are no other subjective symptoms whatever except an occasional light itching sensation. Their course of development is slow. Sometimes these warts may (also) disappear of their own accord.

Treatment

Internal Medication

In order to clear heat, subdue yang, and soften the hard, administer Magnetitum (*Ci Shi*), Concha Margaritiferae (*Zhen Zhu Mu*),

Haematitum (*Dai Zhe Shi*), and raw Concha Ostreae (*Sheng Mu Li*), 30g @, and Flos Carthami Tinctorii (*Hong Hua*), Semen Pruni Persicae (*Tao Ren*), Squama Manitis Pentadactylis (*Chuan Shan Jia*), Spina Gleditschiae Chinensis (*Zao Ci*), Flos Lonicerae Japonicae (*Jin Yin Hua*), and Cortex Phellodendri (*Huang Bai*), 9g @. If the warts occur on the lower limbs, add Radix Achyranthis Bidentatae (*Niu Xi*), 9g. If there is pain, add Rhizoma Corydalis Yanhusuo (*Yuan Hu*), 12g. During menstruation, omit the Flos Carthami Tinctorii, Semen Pruni Persicae, and Squama Manitis Pentadactylis. If warts are concentrated on the face, add Folium Mori Albi (*Sang Ye*) and Flos Chrysanthemi Morifolii (*Ju Hua*), 9g @. One course of treatment consists of 15 *ji* or packets (of the above).

An alternative approach is to take a decoction of Folium Isatidis (*Da Qing Ye*), Radix Isatidis Seu Baphicacanthi (*Ban Lan Gen*), and raw Semen Coicis Lachryma-jobi (*Sheng Yi Ren*), 30g @, and Spica Prunellae Vulgaris (*Xia Gu Cao*) and Radix Gentianae Scabrae (*Long Dan Cao*), 15g @. Reboil the dregs and use as a wash or to rub the affected area. (As for dietary therapy,) boil raw Semen Coicis Lachryma-jobi (*Sheng Yi Ren*), 30g, with rice and make a medicated or herbal porridge. Eat this porridge every morning on an empty stomach for 30 consecutive days.

External Therapies:

1) Auricular acupuncture: *Shen Men* (Spirit Gate) and *Fei Xue* (Lung Pt.) should be needled bilaterally. Press needles should be fixed in the ear with adhesive tape and left in place for from 7-14 days. The patient should be instructed to press (the needles) slightly once per day.

2) Acupuncture: Insert needles at *Gu Kong,* located on the dorsal aspect of the first and second joints of the thumb and also similar points on the big toes. They should be needled to a depth of 5-6 mm. with even supplementation and drainage. The needles should be retained 10 minutes and (a course of treatment is) 10 treatments.

3) The same treatments as for common warts (may be tried).

3. Infectious Soft Warts
Chuan Ran Xing Ruan You

Pathogenesis and pathophysiology: Another name for this condition is *shu ru* (rat's nipple). Its pathogenesis is similar to flat warts, (*i.e.*, according to modern Western medicine,) viral vegetation.

Diagnosis: This condition tends to occur in children. Areas such as the body trunk, the four limbs, and the face and neck are all likely to be affected. Quite often such warts appear in groups, each grouping composed of several warts. They appear as pustules the same color as the skin and vary in size from a grain of rice to a soybean. Their surface is usually smooth and bright with a pit at their center. When their top surface is pricked, a kind of whitish substance may be squeezed out.

Treatment

Puncture the top of the warts and squeeze out the whitish substance before applying *Jui Yi Dan* which is composed of extremely finely powdered prepared Gypsum Fibrosum (*Shi Gao*), 90g, and mercuric oxide, 10g.

4. Filiform Warts
Si Zhuan You

Pathogenesis and pathophysiology: Another name for this condition is *xian hou* (thready warts). (According to modern Western medicine,) it is also a kind of viral vegetation.

Diagnosis: This condition tends to develop on the eyelids and around the neck. It is a kind of tender, filiform growth one millimeter high.

Treatment

Antiwart Powder: Take prepared limestone, (*Chao Shi Tan*) 5g (immerse the limestone in water and fry with a mild fire the filtered sediments until they turn slightly yellowish), powdered Os Draconis (*Long Gu*), Procaine powder, and Borneolum Syntheticum (*Bing Pian*), 30g @. Mix together and grind into a fine powder and apply to the warts. Rub the warts repeatedly with the thumb. Tear off the warts when they feel like they are coming loose.

5. Plantar Warts
Zhe You

Pathogenesis and pathophysiology: (According to modern Western medicine,) this is a kind of viral vegetation.

Diagnosis: Plantar warts tend to occur on the sole of the foot or between the toes. They are the size of a soybean or larger. Because they are a type of keratosis, their surface is often rough and uneven. When their superficial cornification is removed, the deep papillary corneal layer is whitish in color when exposed and bleeds easily. Plantar warts may be distributed over an extensive area if there are a number of them. Tenderness is quite obvious.

Treatment

1) Apply modified *Shui Jing Gao* (47) externally.

2) Apply the oil squeezed from Fructus Bruceae Javanicae (*Ya Dan Zi*).

6. Herpes Simplex
Dan Chun Bao Zheng

Pathogenesis and Pathophysiology: Herpes simplex is also called *re qi*

71

chuang (hot qi sores) and results from invasion of the lung and stomach channels by pathogenic wind. (According to modern Western medicine,) a virus is responsible.

Diagnosis: Herpes simplex is commonly found in those with common cold, pneumonia, or other such febrile diseases. (However, otherwise) healthy persons may also be affected. (Once contracted,) this disease relapses easily. This condition tends to focus on the junctures of the skin and the mucous membranes, such as the oral angle, the borders of the lips, and the external genitalia. Herpes may present as densely packed clusters of water blisters. Their base is often slightly red and there may be heat and itching. It typically resolves itself spontaneously after one week.

Treatment

Internal Medication:

In order to clear heat and dispel wind, it is preferable to administer modified *Xin Yi Qing Fei Yin* which is composed of Gypsum Fibrosum (*Shi Gao*), 30g, white Flos Chrysanthemi Morifolii (*Bai Ju Hua*) and Flos Lonicerae Japonicae (*Jin Yin Hua*), 15g @, Folium Eriobatryae (*Pei Pa Ye*), Fructus Forsythiae Suspensae (*Lian Qiao*), Radix Scutellariae Baicalensis (*Huang Qin*), Fructus Gardeniae Jasminoidis (*Zhi Zi*), and Rhizoma Anemarrhenae (*Zhi Mu*), 9g @, and Flos Magnoliae Officinalis (*Xin Yi*), 5g. Decoct with water and take.

External Therapies:

Apply *Jin Huang San* (18) after mixing with cold, boiled water.

7. Herpes Zoster
Dai Zhuan Bao Zheng

Pathogenesis and pathophysiology: This is also called *she chuan chuang* (snake-like cluster sores) or inflammatory ganglionitis encircling the waist. It is primarily caused by liver fire. (According to modern Western medicine,) is it caused by a virus. *The Golden Mirror of Ancestral Medicine* states, "The folk name of this condition is *she chuan chuang*. It may vary in external appearance. It may be wet or damp and it may be red or yellow. It looks like a cluster of beads. Its dry form may look like red clouds. It typically develops unexpectedly and spreads quickly, giving rise to itching and fever due to wind and fire lingering in the liver and heart channels."

Diagnosis: Herpes zoster tends to be distributed along the pathways of the peripheral nerves and is typically focused on only one side. It is especially frequently found on those areas supplied by the intercostal and trigeminal nerves. Its onset is abrupt or may be preceded by (prodromal) pain. It takes the form of clusters of water blisters of varying size whose surface glisten like pearls. Their base is red and extends broadly. The space between the affected areas is normal. Subjective symptoms are pain and heat of variable degree. Adjacent lymph nodes may be found enlarged. This condition may last for from one to two weeks. In some patients, neuralgia may result as a sequela which may persist for 1—2 months.

Treatment

Internal Medication:

In order to clear damp heat from the liver and gallbladder, administer *Long Dan Xie Gan Tang* (39). In case of constipation, raw Radix Et Rhizoma Rhei (*Sheng Da Huang*), 9g, is often added shortly before the decoction is finished cooking. For neuralgia after the herpes lesions have disappeared, decoct in water Concha Margaritiferae (*Zhen Zhu Mu*), raw Concha Ostreae (*Sheng Mu Li*), Dens Draconis (*Long Chi*), Haematitum (*Dai Zhe Shi*), and Magnetitum (*Ci Shi*), 30g @.

Seven

Skin Infections Due to Insects & Parasites

1. Dermatitis caused by Insect Bite
Chong Yao Pi Yan

Pathogenesis and pathophysiology: This condition is caused by toxins due to insect bites or stings by such insects as lice, mosquitos, ticks, bees, and centipedes.

Diagnosis: Such conditions primarily occur on the exposed extremities and present as minor bleeding, papules, and wheals. Punctures may often be seen in the center of each spot. Itching and pain are variable. As for bites by insects with occult wings, they are characterized by linear of strip-like swelling upon which are densely dotted papules, water blisters, and pustules which give rise to sensations of heat and pain.

Treatment

Internal Medication:

In order to clear heat and resolve toxins, decoct Flos Lonicerae Japonicae (*Jin Yin Hua*) and Herba Cum Radice Taraxaci Mongolici (*Pu Gong Ying*), 30g @, and Radix Glycyrrhizae (*Gan Cao*), 15g, in water and take.

External Therapies:

1) Apply *San Huang Xi Ji* (28) externally.

2) Apply *Zhi Yang Ding* (25) externally.

3) After being bitten by bees or centipedes, cup the area in order to suck out the toxins. An alternative is to mix equal portions of powdered Realgar (*Xiong Huang*) and Herba Cum Radice Asari Seiboldi (*Xi Xin*) with cold, boiled water and apply to the affected area.

2. Dermatitis due to Hookworm
Gou Chong Pi Yan

Pathogenesis and pathophysiology: Another name of this condition is *fen du kuai* (fecal toxin papules). (According to modern Western medicine,) it is due to the penetration of the skin by hookworm larvae.

Diagnosis: Most victims of this disease are farmers, especially those engaged in raising vegetables, silkworms, and mulberry trees. (The patient) typically works barefoot in the fields or has come in contact with feces two or three hours before onset (of this disease). The skin lesions mostly affect the ankles and wrists and especially the fingers and toes. Most commonly, the lesions are scattered, puffy papules and one can see the trace of the entrance of the hookworm larvae on the surface of the skin. Two to seven days after infection, bronchial asthma may present. The acidophil leukocyte counts in the blood or sputum may be elevated and hookworm ovae can also be found in the sputum when asthma is present.

Treatment

Internal Medication:

In most cases, internal medication is not necessary. (However,) if fecal examination reveals hookworm larvae, anthelmintics are applicable.

External Therapies:

1) Use *San Huang Xi Ji* (28) externally.

2) *Qing Dai Gao* (20) is for external use only.

3. Schistosomiasis
Dung Wu Xue Xi Chong Wei Ao Pi Yan

Pathogenesis and pathophysiology: Another name for this condition is *ji she feng* (chicken feces dermatitis). (According to modern Western medicine), it is believed to be an allergic reaction upon entry of the human skin by Schistosoma cercariae flukes (excepting Schistoma japonica).

Diagnosis: This condition may occur for from ten to thirty minutes after contact with (contaminated) water. Initially there is an itching sensation in the affected area. This is followed by the appearance of red spots similar to rape seeds in size. After several hours or one day, these red dots may enlarge into edemic papules or the complicated condition of papules and blisters varying in size from mung to soybeans. The affected area, which feels hard in texture, is either light or bright red. The papules or mixture of papules and blisters may be either densely or sparsely distributed in irregular shaped (patterns). The areas most frequently attacked are the anterior aspect of the calf, and the hands and forearms. Those areas which sink into the soil will not, as a rule, be affected. This condition is characterized by severe itching and lancinating pain which comes to a climax three or four days (after infection) and subsides after one week or so. In recurrent cases, the condition (tends) to be more serious and its course of development prolonged.

Treatment

Internal medication is not necessary in most cases.

External Therapies:

1) *San Huang Xi Ji* (28) may be used externally.

2) *Qing Dai Gao* (20) may be used externally.

3) A mixture of *Jin Huan San* (18), 40g, and petroleum jelly, 100g, can be applied externally.

4) Dissolve Menthol (*Bo He Nao*) and Borneolum Syntheticum (*Bing Pian*), 5g @, in 100ml of 90% alcohol and add phenol, 3g, and 25ml of 15% filtrated Alumen (*Bai Fan*) solution. Use externally when this turns to a milky white suspension.

5) Boil Rhizoma Belamcandae (*She Gan*), 750g, for one hour in 1300 ml of water to which 120g salt should be added after the solution is filtered. Wash the affected area 2 times per day after the solution has been warmed to from 30 - 40 °C.

4. Scabies
Jie Chuang

Pathogenesis and pathophysiology: This condition is primarily caused by the invasion of mites and is complicated by wind, dampness, and hot toxins. *The Golden Mirror of Ancestral Medicine* states, "Scabies are caused by infection. All forms of scabies may start from the webs of the fingers before extending to the rest of the body. The severity of the itching is beyond description."

Diagnosis: This condition is preceded by contact or a history of infection which tends to recur in winter. The webs of both sides of the fingers are mostly stricken. The wrists, axillae or anterior aspect of the armpits, the lower abdomen, and the interior aspect of the thighs are also likely to be attacked. In infants, the palms, finger webs, and even the face may be involved. Those who often wash their hands while working may free their hands from scabies. The primary lesions are within the derma which can curve and extend for two millimeters. There may also be papules and pin-head sized water blisters. Because of intense itching, the patient finds it impossible to refrain from scratching. (However,) this gives rise to secondary, pustular infections and even nephritis. If newly developed water blisters are pricked and the underlying tissues are scraped lightly or if a grayish point is ripped off, tiny, shiny, living dots can be observed with the naked eyes. When placed upon slides, the mites can be seen with microscopic enlargement. If the mites are pricked (i.e. killed), (microscopic examination) will reveal their remains.

Treatment

Internal Medication:

In order to dispel wind, clear heat, and eliminate dampness, decoct Herba Seu Flos Schizonepetae Tenuifoliae (*Jing Jie Sui*), Folium Mori Albi (*Sang Ye*), Radix Sophorae Flavescentis (*Ku Shen*), Cortex Phellodendri (*Huang Bai*), Flos Lonicerae Japonicae (*Jin Yin Hua*), Fructus Forsythiae Suspensae (*Lian Qiao*), Cortex Radicis Moutan (*Mu Dan*), Fructus Kochiae (*Di Fu Zi*), and Rhizoma Dioscoreae Hypoglaucae (*Bi Xie*), 10g @, in water and take.

External Therapies:

1) Bathe in medicated water made from Fructus Zanthoxyli Bungeani (*Chuan Jiao*) and Fructus Kochiae (*Di Fu Zi*), 30g @, or take a warm bath with soap before changing into clean clothes. The affected area should be scrubbed with a 10-20% sulphur paste 2 times per day in the morning and evening for 3 to 4 days. Afterwards one should not bathe or change their clothes (during these three days).

2) Smash the flesh of Semen Hydnocarpi (*Da Feng Zi*) and add an equal amount of unheated petroleum jelly. Apply this mixture to the affected area 3 times per day.

3) "Apply a mixture of smashed Radix Rumicis Crispi (*Yang Ti Gen*) and lard with a bit of salt for better results," according to *Emergency Prescriptions*.

4) According to *Chuan Ya Wai Bian*, "Powder finely Semen Momordicae Cochinensis (*Mu Bei Zi*), 9g, Realgar (*Xiong Huang*), 6g, and Sulphur (*Liu Huang*), 3g, and mix with prepared moxa wool, 90g. Roll into 4 slivers. Fumigate (the body) by placing the slivers on a tile. The cover the body with a quilt (over the smoking tile).

5) *Qing Dai Gao* (20) can be used for secondary infections.

5. Pediculosis
Shi Bin

Pathogenesis and pathophysiology: This is called *shi chuang* (lice lesion) in the classics. It is caused by lice bites, such as head lice, cloth (i.e. body) lice, and crabs.

Diagnosis: This condition manifests as itching or secondary lesions due to scratching, such as scratches, bloody scabs, pigmentation, and pyoderma. Lice or lice eggs may by detected.

Treatment

In most cases, internal medication is not necessary.

External Therapies:

1) Use externally a 5% tincture of Radix Stemonae (*Bai Bu*).

2) Use externally *Zhi Yang Tang* (25).

3) *Yin Xin Wu You San*: Hydrargyrum (*Shui Yin*), prepared with lead, Calomelas (*Qing Fen*), Semen Pruni Armeniacae (*Xing Ren*), peeled

and smashed, Herba Aloes (*Lu Hui*), Realgar (*Xiong Huang*), and Radix Euphorbiae Pallasii (*Lang Du*), 10g @, and Secretio Moschis Moschiferi (*She Xiang*), 1g. The above ingredients should be ground into a fine powder except for the first two. The powders should be sieved and mixed with the Hydrargyrum (*Shui Yin*) and crushed Calomelas (*Qing Fen*). Wash the affected area with medicated water made from Rhizoma Acori Graminei (*Shi Chang Pu*). Then the above mixture should be mixed with cold water (and applied externally).

Eight

Leprosy
Ma Feng

Pathogenesis and pathophysiology: Leprosy is called *lai feng* (*lai* wind). It is caused by invasion of the blood vessels after exposure to epidemic pestilential qi. (According to modern Western medicine,) *Mycobacterium leprae* are found to be the pathogenic bacteria.

Diagnosis: *Mycobacterium leprae* typically invade the peripheral nerves. Sense loss or numbness may be noted in the early stage because of the (subsequent) impairment of the peripheral nerve endings. Therefore, leprosy should be suspected in those with skin conditions characterized by numbness but without pain or itching, such as erythema, leukoderma, and plaques and nodulation.

1) Tuberculoid type: Patients are frequently found to have had contact (with infected individuals) or have a history of living in epidemic areas. The lesions occur on the face, hips, and four extremities. In most cases, only one side of the body is affected. The lesions are macules and papules follicularis in circular and plaque forms with distinct borders. The nerves may be involved in the early stage. (Therefore,) the senses of warmth, pain, and touch may all be diminished in those whose case history extends over one year. Inevitably, the great auricular nerve, the nervus ulnaris, the nervus peroneus communis become thicker and hardened wherever tender spots are found. In the advanced stage, all sorts of deformities, such as facial paralysis or lagophthalmos, or nutritional disturbances, such as ulceration of vesicles and absorption of the phalanges, are common. Dry skin, anhydrosis, and hair loss may result due to atrophy of the sebaceous glands, sweat glands and hair follicles. If the

83

condition only involves the nerves and not the skin, it is considered a purely neurological disorder (not a dermatological one). The lesions may not involve the mucosa, lymph nodes, eyeballs, and other internal organs after the reactional stage. Bacterial examination may be negative (except in the reactional stage), but the lepromin test is typically positive. Pathologically, typical tubercular granuloma is found on further testing.

2) Lepromatous type: (As above,) patients have a history of exposure to leprosy or have lived in a leprotic epidemic area. The skin lesions focus on the face, chest, back, and four extremities symmetrically and systemically. Macules, plaque, nodulation, and diffuse infiltration are common. Diffuse infiltration (here) refers to (a condition) with a shiny surface without distinct border, which turns into leontiasis easily during the last stage. Impairment of the nerves does not develop as early as in the tuberculoid type. Therefore, numbness and the enlargement of the nerves may be absent in the early stage of this type. (The affected area) will not feel as hard initially as in the tuberculoid type. (However,) it likewise will become hardened during the late stage and gives rise to the same lesions to the nerves described above. Accompanying symptoms often include falling of the eyebrows and hair. Likewise, the mucosae and lymph nodes are often involved. In the late stage, the eyes, testes, ovaries, and internal organs, such as the liver and spleen, are also affected. Skin tests (for *Mycobacterium leprae*) are positive even in the early stage even though lepromin tests may be negative. Pathological findings reveal pathogenic bacteria and granuloma derived from *Mycobacterium leprae*.

3) Indeterminate type: (Again, the patient) has either had contact with someone with leprosy or has lived in an epidemic area. (In this case,) the only skin lesions are light colored macules, the borders of which may be either distinct or obscure. There is partial or complete loss of sensitivity in the affected area. (Pathological) changes of the nervous (system) are mild. Skin tests are often negative or show only a weak positive. (However,) the majority of lepromin tests are positive and only a small number (of patients) are (lepromin) negative. Pathological findings are simple, chronic inflammation which may last for years, with most cases (eventually) becoming tuberculoid. The number of cases (which transform into) the lepromatous type are a minority.

4) Dimorphous type: The patient shares similarities with both the lepromatous and tuberculoid types. The skin test is positive and the nasal mucosa test (for *Mycobacterium leprae*) is negative in most cases. Pathological examination often reveals (the existence of) *Mycobacterium leprae* and tubercular granuloma at the same time. If it is not promptly treated, it will often become lepromatous.

Treatment

Internal Medication:

In order to activate the blood and dispel wind, administer *Shao Feng Wan* which are composed of Semen Hydnocarpi (*Da Feng Zi*), fried to remove the oil, 1725g, Rhizoma Atractylodis (*Cang Zhu*), Radix Praeparatus Aconiti Carmichaeli (*Fu Zi*), Ramulus Cinnamomi (*Gui Zhi*), Radix Angelicae Sinensis (*Dang Gui*), Radix Gentianae Macrocephalae (*Qin Jiao*), Radix Angelicae (*Bai Zhi*), Radix Aconiti (*Cao Wu*), Radix Clematidis (*Wei Ling Xian*), Rhizoma Ligustici Wallichii (*Chuan Xiong*), Ramulus Uncariae Cum Uncis (*Gou Teng*), Fructus Chaenomelis Lagenariae (*Mu Gua*), Semen Cuscutae (*Tu Si Zi*), Cortex Cinnamomi (*Rou Gui*), Radix Achyranthis Bidentatae (*Niu Xi*), Radix Polygoni Multiflori (*He Shou Wu*), Rhizoma Homalamenae (*Qian Nian Jian*), mica schist (*Zhu Shi*), Radix Aconiti (*Chuan Wu*), immerse in water to peel the skin, and Radix Ledebouriellae Sesloidis (*Fang Feng*), 120g @, Herba Seu Flos Schizonepetae Tenuifoliae (*Jing Jie Sui*) and raw Semen Coicis Lachryma-jobi (*Sheng Yi Ren*), soaked in water, 240g @, and Agkistroden Seu Bungarus (*Bai Hua She*), 30g. Powder, then pill. Adults should take 6g the first time and increase the dosage 2g each time, 2 times per day (for eight days).

After 8 days, the patient should take 10g of these pills each time, 3 times per day. They should be taken before meals with tea made from stale tea leaves.

(An alternative formulae is) *Bi Sheng San* (which consists of) Radix et Rhizoma Rhei (*Da Huang*), Semen Arecae Catechu (*Bing Lang*), and white Semen Pharbitidis (*Bai Qian Niu Zi*), 3g @, and Calomelas (*Qing Fen*), 5g. Grind into a fine powder and mix thoroughly. Those in robust health should take (this amount in) 5 (equal) doses (for one day's medication). Those who are middle-aged and in poor health due to protracted illness should take it in seven doses with water, (the last dose) being taken before bed.

External Therapies:

1) *Ku Shen Tang* (30) can be used to wash the ulcerous area.

2) *Sheng Ji Gao* (2) or smashed Radix Euphorbiae Pallasii (*Lang Du*) can be used externally for leprotic ulcerations.

Nine

Syphilis
Mei Du

Pathogenesis and pathophysiology: This is called *yang mei chuang* (red bayberry lesion). It is caused by the invasion of evil qi. (According to modern Western medicine,) syphilitic spirochetes are responsible. Two pathways for infection are (known). Direct contact or contraction through sexual activity is called acquired syphilis. The second pathway of infection is called fetal or congenital syphilis. (In this case,) a pregnant woman passes the spirochetes to the fetus from (her) blood stream to the placenta and (hence) to the (baby's) umbilical cord.

Diagnosis: (During) the first stage, hard chancres (develop) after an approximate three week incubation period after sex. A nodulation will appear on the external genitalia which is soybean sized and cherry red with a relatively distinct border. Although painless and itchless, its surface is ulcerous. (In addition,) local lymph nodes may be found swollen at the early stage. Spirochete test is positive and serous tests turn positive during the later stage.

Syphilis of the second stage (can be further divided as follows):

1) Primary second stage syphilis may occur ten weeks after contraction. It manifests as symmetrical and widespread macules, papules, follicular papules, or pustular vesicles. (At this stage,) the mucosae are involved and serum tests show a strong positive.

2) Recurrent second stage syphilis may occur between primary (second stage) syphilis and the next four years (in which) the lesions

are similar to that of the primary type. (However,) the difference is that the lesion is sparsely localized to a particular area, such as the palms or soles. Serum tests indicate a strong positive.

3) In latent second stage syphilis, there may be no symptoms except the positive nature of the serum.

Tertiary Syphilis: Syphilis at this stage affects not only the skin but also (potentially) any other organs and tissues. It jeopardizes one's life when the cardiovascular or nervous systems are involved.

1) Tertiary skin lesions: Typical skin lesions include syphiloma and nodulation. The latter is often scattered in clusters arranged in a circular, curved, or serpiginous manner. If there is ulceration, its margins are noticeably rough and indented. In 70% of cases, serum reaction is positive.

2) Tertiary mucosal lesions: Lesions present in the form of perforations of the nasal septum and both the hard and soft palates and also destroy the uvula.

3) Tertiary bone lesions: Syphilis at this stage may lead to arthritis, the pain of which is aggravated at night and is alleviated by exercise. The pain in this case is non-mobile (i.e. fixed). Periostitis, osteitis gammatus tumidus, and osteomyelitis may also present.

4) Tertiary ocular lesions: These include corneal metritis and iridocyclitis, etc.

5) Tertiary cardiovascular lesions: These include syphilitic aortitis, aortic aneurysm, and aortic incompetence.

6) Tertiary neurological lesions: (Syphilis at this stage may also) give rise to myelopore, general paresis, and tabies dorsalis. Cerebrospinal fluid examination reveals an elevation of cells and protein. Wasserman tests are also positive.

7) Benign tertiary or late benign syphilis: (Diagnosis is based) on a history of venereal disease as revealed by positive serum tests in spite of the absence of signs and symptoms.

Congenital syphilis: The diagnosis (of this type of syphilis) is based on parental history of venereal disease, maternal miscarriage (after four month's pregnancy), premature delivery, and fetal death. Clinical tests, such as bone x-rays, serum reactivity, and cerebral spinal fluid tests (are also helpful). The characteristics of early stage congenital syphilis include wrinkled skin, resemblance of the face to that of an aged person, Hutchinson's teeth, increase of nasal excreta, dark red plaques around the oral and anal orifices, systemically enlarged lymph nodes, enlargement of the liver and spleen, periostitis of the os longum, and positive Wasserman's and Kolmer's serum tests. The characteristics of late stage congenital syphilis are intestinal keratitis, a high palantine arc, overgrowth of the medial end of the right clavicle, and thin tibia. Other symptoms may include neurological deafness, saddle nose, etc.

Treatment

Internal Medication:

In order to resolve toxins and eliminate dampness:

1) *San Xian Dan He Ji: San Xian Dan* (a patent medicine), 2.56g, Cortex Phellodendri (*Huang Bai*), 5.12g, and Radix Glycyrrhizae (*Gan Cao*), 2.56g. The above ingredients should be ground into a fine powder and mixed together thoroughly before being made into forty pills with water. The accompanying 2 bowls of water should be made from Rhizoma Smilacis Glabrae (*Tu Fu Ling*), 30g. If (the patient desires) to take as powder instead of as pills, the powder can be wrapped in bananas, glutinous rice, sweet potatoes, longan pulp, or vegetable leaves so as to avoid irritation of the oral cavity. One course of treatment consists of 20 days.

2) *Tu Fu Ling He Ji:* Rhizoma Smilacis Glabrae (*Tu Fu Ling*), 60g, Flos Lonicerae Japonicae (*Jin Yin Hua*) and Fructus Xanthii (*Cang Er Zi*), 15g @, Radix Clematidis (*Wei Ling Xian*) and Cortex Cynanchi Atrati (*Bai Wei*), 9g @, and Radix Glycyrrhizae (*Gan Cao*), 6g. Boil the above in 800 ml water until reduced to 400 ml. One packet or *ji* per day should be taken 3 times per day with meals. One course of treatment consists of 60 consecutive days.

External Therapies:

Ulcerations due to hard chancre, second stage syphilis, and skin rupture and rupture of congenital syphilis can be treated with *E Huang San,* which is composed of powdered Semen Phaseoli Munginis (*Lu Dou Fen*), 30g, Calomelas (*Qing Fen*) and Cortex Phellodendri (*Huang Bai*), 10g @, and aged Pollen Pini (*Song Hua Fen*) and powdered Talcum (*Hua Shi Fen*), 15g @. The above ingredients should be ground into a fine powder which then can be mixed with roasted sesame oil (*Xiang You*) before applying to the affected areas.

As for ulcerous conditions due to tertiary stage syphiloma and nodulation, first administer *Wu Wu Dan,* (which consists of) powdered, prepared Gypsum Fibrosum (*Shu Shi Gao*) and mercuric oxide (*Sheng Dan*), etc., in equal portions in order to evacuate the pus and eliminate necrotic tissue. This should then be followed by external application of *Sheng Ji Gao* (21) in order to astringe and generate new tissue.

Ten _____

Neurological Skin Disorders

1. Neurodermatitis
Shen Jing Xing Pi Yan

Pathogenesis and pathophysiology: This is called *niu pi xian* (ox skin tinea) in the classics. It is caused by malnutrition of the skin due to insufficiency of the *ying* and blood and disturbance of wind and dryness resulting from blood vacuity. Because it is a neurotic manifestation, it can be induced by emotional disturbances and distress, neurasthenia, local friction and irritation by one's collar, or by scratching.

Diagnosis: Typically the patient has a history of allergies, such as urticaria and dermographism. Sour and spicy foods or localized irritation may also be precipitating factors. Such conditions tend to localize in areas exposed to frequent friction, such as the neck which accounts for over 90% of cases. (Next, in descending order of frequency come the) sacrum, exterior surfaces of the four limbs, interiors of the thighs, scrotum, and perineum. Occasionally it may be found distributed symmetrically. The preceding symptom is itching which is so severe (that one cannot refrain from) scratching. Pin-head sized, flat papules in irregular, triangular, or multi-angular shapes may appear. (Such papules feel) dry and firm and rapidly develop lichenoid plaques.

Treatment

Internal Medication:

In order to nourish the blood, dispel wind, and moisten dryness, administer *Si Wu Xiao Feng Tang*. (It is comprised of) raw Semen Coicis Lachryma-jobi (*Sheng Yi Ren*) and Concha Margaritiferae (*Zhen Zhu Mu*), 30g @, dried Radix Rehmanniae (*Gan Di Huang*), and Cortex Radicis Dictamni (*Bai Xian Pi*), 15g @, and Radix Angelicae Sinensis (*Dang Gui*), Rhizoma Ligustici Wallichii (*Chuan Xiong*), Radix Rubrus Paeoniae Lactiflorae (*Chi Shao*), Radix Ledebouriellae Sesloidis (*Fang Feng*), Herba Seu Flos Schizonepetae Tenuifoliae (*Jing Jie Sui*), and Fructus Schizandrae Chinensis (*Wu Wei Zi*), 10g @. Decoct with water and take.

External Therapies:

1) Apply externally a 20% tincture of Radix Stemonae (*Bai Bu*).

2) Use a moderately warm compress made from a decoction of Radix Sophorae Flavescentis (*Ku Shen*) and Herba Artemisiae Capillaris (*Yin Chen Hao*), 30g @, and Retinervus Fructi Luffae (*Si Gua Luo*), 50g.

3) Prick the affected area with a plum blossom needle every day. Ten treatment constitute 1 course.

4) Vinegar and egg: Take 3 eggs and 500g black vinegar. Immerse the eggs in the black vinegar for one week. Then remove and crack. Apply (the insides) externally after whipping them into a paste.

5) Fumigation therapy (32)

6) *Zhi Yang Ding* (25) may be applied externally.

2. Pruritus
Yang Zheng

Pathogenesis and pathophysiology: This is also called *yang zheng* (itching condition) in the classics. It is caused by wind and dryness due to blood vacuity and hyperactivity of the liver or the downward percolation of damp heat (derived from) liver fire. (According to modern Western medicine,) systemic pruritus is often associated with climatic dryness, dryness and atrophy of the skin due to old age, disorders of the endocrine (system), diabetes, jaundice, and hematological disease. Senile pruritus and seasonal pruritus fall into this category. (Whereas,) localized pruritus is frequently caused by localized friction or irritation, insect bite, hemorrhoids, trichomoniasis, pinworm, and leukorrhea, such as in pruritus vulvae, perianal pruritus, and scrotal pruritus.

Diagnosis: The skin condition is preceded by itching. Fingernail marks and bloody scabs may appear after scratching. In severe cases, folliculitis, furuncles, and eczematous dermatitis may accompany. (Pruritus is characterized by) paroxysms of severe itching which are often aggravated after drinking alcohol, before bed, after a bath, and during sleep when the quilt is (too) warm. (Pruritus) is also related to emotional disturbance. Victims will scratch until the skin bleeds.

Treatment

Internal Medication:

In order to facilitate the production of fluids and humor, moisten dryness, and stop itching, *Run Fu Tang* (11) (is indicated). *Long Dan Xie Gan Tang* (39) is applicable for scrotal itching and pruritus of the female genitalia.

External Therapies:

1) Apply externally a 20% tincture of Radix Stemonae (*Bai Bu*).

93

2) Acupuncture: Pruritus of the four limbs and body trunk can be treated by *Qu Chi* (LI 11), *He Gu* (LI 4), *Xue Hai* (Sp 10), and *Zu San Li* (St 36). *Qu Gu* (CV 2) and *Chang Qiang* (GV 1) can be used for perineal and perianal pruritus.

3) For systemic pruritus, wash with *Ku Shen Tang* (30). For perianal pruritus, wash with a decoction made from Radix Sophorae Flavescentis (*Ku Shen*) and Herba Artemesiae Capillaris (*Yin Chen Hao*), 30g @. For pruritus vulvae, wash with a decoction made from Herba Spirodelae Seu Lemnae (*Fu Ping*), Fructus Kochiae (*Di Fu Zi*), and Fructus Xanthii (*Cang Er Zi*), 30g @. For scrotal itching, wash with a soup made from Retinervus Fructi Luffae (*Si Gua Luo*) and Folium Artemesiae Argyii (*Ai Ye*), 30g @, and Realgar (*Xiong Huang*) and Fructus Zanthoxyli Bungeani (*Chuan Jiao*), 10g @.

4) Apply externally *Zhi Yang Ding* (25).

3. Nodular Prurigo
Jie Xing Yang Zheng

Pathogenesis and pathophysiology: This condition is probably associated with insect bites. Some (authorities) consider it a special type of nodular neurodermatitis. Most victims are adult females.

Diagnosis: (This condition) tends to focus on the four extremities and especially around the anterior aspect of the calf. The skin erupts in the form of substantial, semispheric nodulations, dark brown in color and the size of (soy) beans. The surface (of the skin) feels dry and rough. There is severe itching. This condition is chronic with a high incidence of recurrence.

Treatment

Internal Medication:

In order to eliminate dampness, resolve toxins, activate the blood, and dispel stasis, decoct in water and take Radix Sophorae Flavescentis (*Ku Shen*), Flos Immaturus Sophorae Japonicae (*Huai Hua*), Fructus Tribuli Terrestris (*Bai Ji Li*), Cortex Radicis Dictamni (*Bai Xian Pi*), Radix Angelicae Sinensis (*Dang Gui*), and Radix Salviae Miltior-rhizae (*Dan Shen*), 15g @, and Fructus Forsythiae Suspensae (*Lian Qiao*), Radix Gentianae Scabrae (*Long Dan Cao*), Cortex Radicis Moutan (*Dan Pi*), and Radix Ledebouriellae Sesloidis (*Fang Feng*) 10g @.

External Therapies:

1) Apply externally a 20% tincture of Radix Stemonae (*Bai Bu*).

2) Use externally *Zhi Yang Ding* (25).

Eleven

Physically Induced Dermatoses

1. Clavus (Corns)
Ji Yan

Pathogenesis and pathophysiology: These are also called *rou ci* (flesh thorns). They are caused by frequent friction, constant pressure, inappropriate shoe size, prolonged walking, or clubfoot.

Diagnosis: (Corns) occur in areas that are rubbed and pressed such as the sole, the borders of the sole, and between the toes. The (subsequent) lesions is a cone-like overgrowth of a horny layer whose base protrudes and stands in relief. Its tip points to the mammillary layer of the dermis, which thus causes marked tenderness. If corns develop between the toes, the skin often appears wet and fragile.

Treatment

1) Grind equal portions of Cortex Radicis Lycii (*Di Gu Pi*) and Flos Carthami Tinctorii (*Hong Hua*) into powder, mix and make into a paste with roasted sesame oil and flour. Before applying externally, peel away the hardened skin over the affected area. Change the dressing every other day.

2) Acupuncture: Insert a 28 ga. stainless steel needle into the center of the corn to a depth of from 1 to 1.5 *cun* until it bleeds. One acupuncture treatment will, as a rule, suffice. But in severe cases, treat once per week. Five or six consecutive treatments should relieve the symptoms.

3) Apply externally *Shui Jing Gao* (47).

2. Callus
Pian Zhi

Pathogenesis and pathophysiology: This condition is a protective response to longterm mechanical friction.

Diagnosis: (Callosities) are characterized by localized thickening of the horny layer of the epidermis with obscure borders. Their surface feels smooth and substantial. In most cases, there are no subjective symptoms. Callosities tend to develop on the protrusions of the palms and soles.

Treatment

Pian Zhi Gao, (which) is composed of raw limestone and caustic natrium, 90g @, soap, 45g, and powdered Camphora (*Zhang Nao*), 10g, may be applied after being made into a paste with water.

3. Chapping of the hands and feet
Shou Zu Jun Lie

Pathogenesis and pathophysiology: This is called *jun lie chuang* (cracked lesion) in the classics. It is caused by injury to the palms or soles, such as friction, pressure, wounds, and immersion.

Diagnosis: (This condition) tends to focus on the surface of the palms, the fingertips, or lateral edges of the hands, feet, or heels. The lesion often causes cracks of varied depths and lengths in the above areas. The thicker the skin, the deeper the cracks. These may cause bleeding and pain. Most cases are found in winter.

Treatment

1) *Gan Gao You* (27) can be used externally.

2) Wash with a decoction of Cortex Radicis Lycii (*Di Gu Pi*) and Alum (*Ku Fan*), 30g @.

3) Heat a small piece of beeswax with a little sesame oil until the wax melts. Drip this into the cracks while still warm.

4) *Run Ji Gao* (32) can be applied externally.

4. Miliaria Rubra (Prickly Heat)
Hong She Li Zheng

Pathogenesis and pathophysiology: This is called *fei cuo chuang* (miliaria acne lesion) in the classics and *fei zi* (miliaria) amongst the people. It is caused by an accumulation of summer dampness in the surface and impeded perspiration due to high temperature and humidity during the summer. Li Yan, (a distinguished TCM practitioner of the Ming Dynasty) states in the *Yi Xue Ru Men* (*Entering the Gate of Medicine*, 1624 CE), "Miliaria develops because of heavy humidity upon perspiration. In mild cases, the condition looks like millet...In severe cases, extensive ulceration arises from profuse sweat." In his *Shi She Mi Lu* (*Secret Record of the Star Chamber*), Chen Shi-duo of the Qing Dynasty states, "Miliaria appears as a result of the complication of (pathogenic) summer qi with heat."

Diagnosis: (Miliaria) is characterized by sudden onset. It tends to develop around the forehead, neck, chest, back, and cubital creases, or (at least) those areas are more extensively affected. The lesions consist of densely spotted papules or papulo-vesicles the size of pin heads. Moderate redness may appear. Burning and itching are often felt subjectively.

Treatment

Internal Medication:

In order to clear summerheat and scatter heat, *Lu Dou Tang* is recommended. Boil 50g of Semen Phaseoli Munginis (*Lu Dou*) and then add Herba Menthae (*Bo He*), 10g, and sugar. (This beverage can be taken) as a substitute for tea.

External Therapies:

1) (A mixture of) powdered Talcum (*Hua Shi Fen*), 30g, and powdered Semen Phaeoli Minginis (*Lu Dou Fen*), 15g, can be dusted over the affected area after bathing.

2) Bath in medicated water made from Talcum (*Hua Shi*), 180g, and Radix Glycyrrhizae (*Gan Cao*), 30g.

3) Rub externally (the affected areas) with sliced cucumber or the juice of smashed fresh leaves of the towel gourd.

5. Frostbite
Dong Chuang

Pathogenesis and pathophysiology: Another name for this condition is *dong zhu* (frozen lump). It is caused by stasis and stagnation of qi and blood due to invasion by pathogenic cold. (According to modern Western medicine,) it is a chronic infiltration of the local tissues due to impeded blood circulation.

Diagnosis: The initial lesions take the form of localized masses or plaques ranging in size from broad beans to coins with a red border surrounding a greenish purple center. Water blisters may appear leading to ulceration after the blisters rupture. (This condition) typically occurs symmetrically at the tips of the extremities and especially on the dorsal aspect of the hand, the edges of the soles, the lower limbs, cheeks, and auricles. Subjectively, there is itching which is aggravated by warmth.

Treatment

Internal Medication:

In order to move the qi and nourish the blood, use *Ren Shen Yang Yong Tang* which is composed of Radix Codonopsis Pilosulae (*Dang Shen*) and Radix Astragali Membranacei (*Huang Qi*), 15g @, Sclerotium Poriae Cocoris (*Fu Ling*) and Radix Albus Paeoniae Lactiflorae (*Bai Shao*), 12g @, Ramulus Cinnamomi (*Gui Zhi*), Rhizoma Atractylodis Macrocephalae (*Bai Zhu*), and Radix Praeparatus Glycyrrhizae (*Zhi Gan Cao*), 9g @, Radix Coquitus Rehmanniae (*Shu Di*), 24g, and Fructus Schizandrae Chinensis (*Wu Wei Zi*) and Radix Polygalae Tenuifoliae (*Yuan Zhi*), 3g @. Decoct with water and take. To warm the channels and scatter cold, *Dang Gui Si Ni Tang* (4) may be administered.

External Therapies:

1) During the first stage of skin reddening, wash with moderately warm water made from Fructus Chaenomelas Lagenariae (*Mu Gua*) and pepper (*La Jiao*), 30g @, and scallion (*Cong*), 60g.

2) During the water blister stage, apply a mixture of honey (*Feng Mi*), 70g, and lard (*Zhu You*), 30g.

3) During the ulcerous stage, mix powdered Fructificatio Lasiopherae (*Ma Bo*), 20g and petroleum jelly, 80g; or apply *Sheng Ji Gao* (21).

4) In mild cases, *Hong Ling Jin* (24) is recommended externally. An alternative is to steam and wash the affected area with 1500ml of medicated water made from Melanteritum (*Qing Fan*), 100g.

6. Summertime Dermatitis
Xia Ling Pi Yan

Pathogenesis and pathophysiology: This condition results from invasion of the skin by spleen dampness and the accumulation of summerheat. (Modern Western medicine believes) that) it is associated with high temperature and irritation by sweat.

Diagnosis: The lesions present symmetrically and tend to focus on the lateral aspects of the four limbs. They mainly manifest as tiny papules which may be followed by bloody scabs and scratch marks. Itching is severe. Often, this condition recurs during the summer each year.

Treatment

Internal Medication:

In order to eliminate dampness and clear summerheat, administer *Qing Huo Yi Ren Tang* (6).

External Therapies:

1) Apply externally *Fu Fang Ku Shen Fen* (33) after mixing with water.

2) *San Huang Xi Ji* (28) may be applied externally.

3) *Zhi Yang Ding* (25) may be used externally.

Twelve

Erythematous Scaly Skin Diseases

1. Psoriasis
Ying Xie Bing

Pathogenesis and pathophysiology: Psoriasis is called *song pi xian* (pine skin tinea). When it appears in dotted form, it is called *bai bi* (white mark). It is caused by wind and dampness due to blood exhaustion in turn due to invasion by pathogenic wind. In *The Golden Mirror of Ancestral Medicine* it is said: "Pine skin tinea is named after the resemblance of the red and white dotted skin to pine tree bark. Itching is constant." Further: "*Bai bi* arises from the dry white skin as itchy macula and scabs. The scaly white skin is due to scratching. (This condition) is caused by malnourishment (of the skin) when blood dryness is caused by attack of the skin by pathogenic wind."

Diagnosis: The lesions tend to develop on the lateral aspects of the four limbs, and especially on the lateral side of the elbows and knees. They may also concentrate on the body trunk and scalp. The lesions are pink or red papules and plaques with distinctive borders. They are characterized by many layers of dry, silverish scales. If (the skin) is lightly scraped by a bamboo sliver, a pink and semi-transparent membrane may be formed (which is called membrane phenomenon). If one keeps on scraping, tiny spots of blood (called petechial hemorrhage) may develop. Lesions may vary in size from dots to coins and may be either circular or geographic in shape. If lesions appear in the scalp they will be dark red in color and will be covered with grayish white scales from which the hair may grow in bundles. However, the hair will not fall out. If the lesions occur on the

103

fingernails or the toenails, they will appear as dotted depressions similar to thimbles used to push sewing needles through cloth.

Treatment

Internal Medication:

During the acute, progressive stage, in order primarily to cool the blood, dispel wind, and nourish the blood, use Radix Rehmanniae (*Sheng Di*), 30g, and Folium Mori Albi (*Sang Ye*), white Flos Chrysanthemi Morifolii (*Bai Ju Hua*), Radix Rubrus Paeoniae Lactiflorae (*Chi Shao*), Cortex Radicis Moutan (*Mu Dan Pi*), Cortex Radicis Dictamni (*Bai Xian Pi*), Radix Sophorae Flavescentis (*Ku Shen*), Fructus Kochiae (*Di Fu Zi*), Fructus Xanthii (*Cang Er Zi*), and Zaocys (*Wu Xiao She*), 10g @. For the static or deteriorating stage, in order to nourish the blood, dispel wind, and moisten dryness, use Radix Coquitus Rehmanniae (*Shu Di*), 30g, Radix Polygoni Multiflori (*He Shou Wu*), 15g, and Radix Angelicae Sinensis (*Dang Gui*), Radix Albus Paeoniae Lactiflorae (*Bai Shao*), Semen Cuscutae (*Tu Si Zi*), Radix Sophorae Flavescentis (*Ku Shen*), Cortex Radicis Dictmani (*Bai Xian Pi*), and Zaocys (*Wu Xiao She*), 10g @. An alternative is to use modified *Gui Zhi Dang Gui Tang* (1).

External Therapies:

1) *Yin Xie Bing Yu Ji* (31)

2) Ointment made of poplar leaves: Place poplar leaves (*Yang Shu Ye*) in a pan and boil with water. Strain and remove the dregs. Then reduce the blackened juice to a sticky ointment which should then be mixed with 30% petroleum jelly.

3) Psoriasis tincture: Sanguis Draconis (*Xue Jie*) and salicylic acid (*Liu Suan*), 5g @, and Camphora (*Zheng Nao*), 2g. Powder and mix with castor oil (*Bi Ma You*), 10g. Then add to 100ml 90% alcohol.

4) Apply externally a 10% sulphur ointment.

2. Nodular Erythema
Jie Xing Hong Ban

Pathogenesis and pathophysiology: This condition is quite similar to what is called *fu yin zhu* (gangrene of the yin aspect) in the classics. It is believed to be caused by obstruction of the channels and Connecting vessels due to invasion of the lower burner by damp heat. (However,) some people believe it is an allergic response to infection. In cases of rheumatic fever, tonsillitis, and tuberculosis, streptococcus and tubercular bacilli may be found responsible (according to Western pathology). In *The Golden Mirror of Ancestral Medicine* it states, "This condition is likely to occur three *cun* above the medial malleolus. Its initial symptoms are reddening of the skin like millet, pain which increases daily, and swelling, redness, and hardness which increase until (the lesion) becomes like an egg. This condition is caused by the accumulation of damp heat in the three yin (channels)."

Diagnosis: This condition is common amongst the young, especially young women and also especially during spring and fall. Lesions tend to occur symmetrically around the anterior aspect of the lower leg in the form of nodulations which are either bright or dark red in color and 1-2 *cun* in diameter. The lesion is raised above the surface of the skin. Pain is experienced subjectively and there are tender spots (to palpation). The color (of the lesion) will not fade upon pressure. As a rule, water blisters and ulcerations will not occur during the course of the disease. (However,) there may be systemic symptoms, such as fever, headaches, arthralgia, fatigue, and loss of appetite. The course of disease may last from 4—6 weeks and may recur.

Treatment

Internal Medication:

In order to clear heat and eliminate dampness, activate the blood and open the connecting vessels, take Radix Rehmanniae (*Sheng Di*), 25g,

Flos Chrysanthemi Morifolii (*Ju Hua*), Herba Cum Radice Taraxaci Mongolici (*Pu Gong Ying*), Fructus Chaenomelis Lagenariae (*Mu Gua*), Caulis Milletiae Seu Spatholobi (*Ji Xue Teng*), and Radix Glycyrrhizae (*Gan Cao*), 15g @, and Folium Mori Albi (*Sang Ye*), Radix Gentianae Macrocephalae (*Qin Jiao*), Rhizoma Atractylodis (*Cang Zhu*), Radix Clematidis (*Wei Ling Xian*), and Radix Angelicae Sinensis (*Dang Gui*), 10g @. Decoct in water and take.

External Therapies:

1) Hot compresses may be made from a decoction of Radix Glycyrrhizae (*Gan Cao*), Lignum Sappanis (*Su Mu*), and Rhizoma Nardostachys (*Gan Song*), 30g @.

2) *Yu Lu San* (26) may be used externally.

3) *Qing Dai Gao* (20) may be used externally.

3. Erythema Multiforme
Duo Xing Hong Ban

Pathogenesis and pathophysiology: This is called *mao yan chuang* (cat's eye lesion) in the literature. It is due to long-standing damp heat in the spleen channel complicated by wind pathogens. (According to modern Western medicine,) this condition is probably an allergic response to infections, such as tonsillitis, and also possibly to (certain) food. *The Golden Mirror of Ancestral Medicine* states: "Frequently (this condition) appears around the face and all over the body due to longterm accumulation of damp heat in the spleen channel complicated by external wind. Its shape during the initial stage is like a cat's eye with shining brightness and incredible itching but without suppuration or bleeding."

Diagnosis: This condition is quite common amongst youth and young adults in the spring and fall. The lesions tend to symmetrically involve the palms, the dorsal aspects of the hands, the soles, the dorsal aspects of the feet, and the forearms. The oral mucosa and external genitalia may also be involved in a minority of cases. The lesions typically present as pleomorphic macules, papules, and water blisters. Also, typically there is dark red or purple at the center of erythema often overlapped by blisters. (In addition,) erythema may also be surrounded by red rings which then resemble an iris. If the oral or labial mucosa are involved, there may be ulcerations of the mouth or lips. The patient may feel burning heat, pain, or itching followed by such systemic symptoms as fever, headache, and arthralgia in varying degrees. Each attack may last 2—3 weeks and relapse is easy.

Treatment

Internal Medication:

In order to cool the blood, clear heat, and eliminate dampness, administer modified *Qing Ji Sheng Shi Tang* composed of Radix Rehmanniae (*Sheng Di*), 30g and Rhizoma Atractylodis (*Cang Zhu*), Radix Glycyrrhizae (*Gan Cao*), Caulis Akebiae Mutong (*Mu Tong*), Rhizoma Alismatis (*Ze Xie*), Rhizoma Cimicifugae (*Sheng Ma*), Rhizoma Atractylodis Macrocephalae (*Bai Zhu*), Fructus Gardeniae Jasminoïdis (*Shan Zhi Zi*), Rhizoma Coptidis Chinensis (*Huang Lian*), Cortex Radicis Moutan (*Dan Pi*), Radix Rubrus Paeoniae Lactiflorae (*Chi Shao*), and Radix Sophorae Flavescentis (*Ku Shen*), 10g @. Decoct with water and take.

External Therapies:

1) Cold compresses can be made from a decoction of Flos Lonicerae Japonicae (*Jin Yin Hua*), Fructus Cnidii Monnieri (*She Chuang Zi*), Radix Sophorae Flavescentis (*Ku Shen*), Fructus Xanthii (*Cang Er Zi*), and Fructus Kochiae (*Di Fu Zi*), 30g @.

2) *Qing Dai Gao* (20) may be used externally.

107

3) For those with ulceration and suppuration, use cold compresses with a decoction made from raw olives or a 10% solution of Radix Glycyrrhizae (*Gan Cao*).

4. Pityriasis Simplex
Dan Chun Kang Zheng

Pathogenesis and pathophysiology: This condition is also called *tao hua xian* (peach flower tinea) or *chong ban* (worm plaque). It is caused by an ascent of wind heat from the lungs and stomach. (According to modern Western medicine,) it might be associated with an intestinal parasite.

Diagnosis: This condition is commonly encountered in school-aged children and is also found among young women. The lesions mainly focus on the face in the form of light colored circular or oval macules which may begin light red in color and become light white later on. Their border is often indistinct. There may also be a little grayish, furfuraceous desquamation. As a rule, there are no subjective symptoms.

Treatment

Internal Medication:

In order to clear heat and dispel wind, administer *Shu Feng Qing Re Yin* which is composed of Flos Lonicerae Japonicae (*Jin Yin Hua*), 15g, Radix Sophorae Flavescentis (*Ku Shen*), Radix Ledebouriellae Sesloidis (*Fang Feng*), and Herba Seu Flos Schizonepetae Tenuifoliae (*Jing Jie Sui*), 9g @, and Buthus Martensis (*Quan Xie*), Periostracum Cicadae (*Chan Tui*), and Spina Gleditschiae Chinensis (*Zao Ci*), 3g @. Decoct with water and take.

External Therapies:

1) Apply externally a 5% sulphur ointment.

2) Use *Pi Zhi Gao* (40) externally.

5. Pityriasis Rosacea
Mei Gui Kang Zheng

Pathogenesis and pathophysiology: Another name for this condition is *mu zi xian* (mother-son tinea). It is caused by blockage of the *cou li* (striae) due to wind heat and blood dryness. (According to modern Western medicine,) it is mild form of acute dermatitis.

Diagnosis: This condition is commonly found among adults in the Spring and Fall. The body trunk and the proximal ends of the four limbs are the most likely to be afflicted. If it occurs on the chest or back, the lesions will parallel the ribs in the form of irregularly oval shaped, rosy macules. Their size may be similar to pumpkin seeds and they are typically characterized by a yellowish spot in their centers. Delicate marks may be noted after scratching. Their narrow border looks pink and is covered by furfuraceous scaling. Larger sized macules may first appear followed by groups of lesions over one to two weeks later. There may be slight itching. This disease is often self-limiting and spontaneous recovery is expected in from 4—6 weeks.

Treatment

Internal Medication:

In order to cool the blood, dispel wind, and clear heat, administer Radix Rehmanniae (*Sheng Di*), 25g, Flos Chrysanthemi Morifolii (*Ju Hua*), Radix Rubrus Paeoniae Lactiflorae (*Chi Shao*), Fructus Gardeniae Jasminoidis (*Shan Zhi Zi*), Radix Sophorae Flavescentis (*Ku Shen*), Cortex Radicis Dictamni (*Bai Xian Pi*), Herba Siegesbeckiae (*Xi Jian Cao*), and Radix Lithospermi Seu Arnebiae (*Hong Tiao Zi Cao*), 10g @, and Periostracum Cicadae (*Chan Tui*) and Radix Glycyrrhizae (*Gan Cao*), 3g @. Decoct with water and take.

External Therapies:

1) *San Huang Xi Ji* (28) may be used externally.

2) *Ku Shen Tang* (30) may be used externally.

Thirteen _____

Vesicular Dermatitis

1. Pemphigus
Tian Bao Chuang

Pathogenesis and pathophysiology: Another name for this condition is
huo chi chuang (flaming red lesion). It is caused by attack of the lung
channel by summerheat and damp heat pathogens and by the
accumulation of heart fire and spleen dampness. *The Golden Mirror
of Ancestral Medicine* states, "This condition is due to hyperactivity
of heart fire which invades the lungs. (The size of the vesicles) may
vary from that of Semen Euryalis Ferocis (*Qian Shi*) to that of
Chinese chess pieces. The condition is characterized by serous blisters
among which are red ones called *huo chi chuang*. Those with red
bases and white tips are called *tian bao chuang*. This condition tends
to spread all over the body accompanied by heat and pain. The
lesions never feel hard even before eruption. (However,) upon
perforation, the toxic fluid does not smell offensively."

Diagnosis:

1. Common Pemphigus: This is common in middle-aged adults. It is
characterized by systemic lesions often involving the oral mucosa.
Various sized, circular or irregularly shaped water blisters may be
found with thin, loose walls resulting in epidermolysis. There is
localized itching and pain accompanied by such systemic symptoms
as fever, loss of appetite, and (general) weakness.

2. Pemphigus Foliaceous: This condition presents as flaccid water
blisters, the fluid of which is often turbid. Grayish yellow scabs are

formed after drying. Because the water blisters develop incessantly and the affected area expands increasingly, it may look like exfoliative dermatitis with continuous scabbing. The excreta beneath the scab has an offensive odor and epidermolysis is more pronounced.

3. Pemphigus Vegetans: The frequently affected areas are the axillae, umbilicus, the peri-anus, and external genitalia. Crusts may form after perforation of the water blisters. Papillary proliferation may occur simultaneously at the base of the lesion. The suppurated excreta smells fetid.

4. Pemphigus Erythematosus: This condition often occurs around the face and on the body trunk. Erythema often precedes the appearance of water blisters, scabs, and scaling.

Treatment

Internal Medication:

(The therapeutic principles for the treatment of pemphigus are) to discharge fire, resolve toxins, and eliminate dampness. If fire is more prominent than dampness, it is preferable to administer *Jie Du Xie Xin Tang* which consists of Gypsum Fibrosum (*Shi Gao*) and Talcum (*Hua Shi*), 30g @, and Radix Scutellariae Baicalensis (*Huang Qin*), Rhizoma Coptidis Chinensis (*Huang Lian*), Fructus Arctii (*Niu Bang Zi*), Radix Anemarrhenae (*Zhi Mu*), Fructus Gardeniae Jasminoidis (*Shan Zhi Zi*), Radix Ledebouriellae Sesloidis (*Fang Feng*), Radix Scrophulariae Ningpoensis (*Xuan Shen*), Herba Seu Flos Schizonepetae Tenuifoliae (*Jing Jie*), Caulis Akebiae Mutong (*Mu Tong*), and Radix Glycyrrhizae (*Gan Cao*), 10g @. Decoct with water and take.

If dampness is more prominent than fire, *Qing Pi Chu Shi Yin* is preferable and includes Herba Artemesiae Capillaris (*Yin Chen Hao*) and Radix Rehmanniae (*Sheng Di*), 30g @, Radix Rubrus Paeoniae Lactiflorae (*Chi Shao*), Rhizoma Atractylodis Macrocephalae (*Bai Zhu*), Rhizoma Atractylodis (*Cang Zhu*), Radix Scutellariae Baicalen-

112

sis (*Huang Qin*), Tuber Ophiopogonis Japonicae (*Mai Men Dong*), Fructus Gardeniae Jasminoidis (*San Zhi Zi*), Rhizoma Alismatis (*Ze Xie*), Radix Glycyrrhizae (*Gan Cao*), Fructus Forsythiae Suspensae (*Lian Qiao*), and Fructus Citri Seu Ponciri (*Zhi Qiao*), 10g @, and Natrii Sulfas Exsiccatus (*Yuan Ming Fen*), 3g taken separately. Decoct with water and take.

External Therapies:

1) *San Huang Xi Ji* (28) may be used externally.

2) Wet compresses may be made from a decoction of Radix Glycyrrhizae (*Gan Cao*) and Radix Scutellariae Baicalensis (*Huang Qin*), 60g @.

3) Dust externally with *Qing Dai San* (20) or *Si Huang San* 19) in cases less productive of fluid.

2. Vesicular Dermatitis
Bao Zheng Yang Pi Yan

Pathogenesis and pathophysiology: This condition develops from an accumulation of damp heat in the muscles and skin.

Diagnosis: This condition often occurs symmetrically around the shoulder, low back, sacrum, hips, and the four limbs. Lesions are multi-shaped water blisters occurring in clusters. The walls of these blisters are relatively thick and do not easily rupture. Erythema, papules, wheals, pustules, and pigmentation may also occur. There is extreme itching and the disease progresses slowly with frequent recurrences.

Treatment

Internal Medication:

In order to clear heat, eliminate dampness, and stop itching, administer modified *Er Miao Tang* composed of Semen Arecae Catechu (*Bing Lang*), Radix Scutellariae Baicalensis (*Huang Qin*), Radix Atractylodis (*Cang Zhu*), Radix Sophorae Flavescentis (*Ku Shen*), Fructus Kochiae (*Di Fu Zi*), Rhizoma Alismatis (*Ze Xie*), and Radix Atractylodis Macrocephalae (*Bai Zhu*), 10g @. Decoct with water and take.

External Therapies:

1) Use *Ku Shen Tang* (30) as an external wash.

2) *San Huang Xi Ji* (28) can be used as an external lotion.

3) *Si Huang San* (19) or *Qing Dai Gao* (20) can be applied externally after being prepared with water.

Fourteen

Collagen Diseases

1. Systemic Lupus Erythematosus
Xi Tong Hong Ban Xing Lang Chuang

Pathogenesis and pathophysiology: This disease is due to an accumulation of heat in the heart and spleen and insufficiency of kidney yin (which gives rise to) hyperactivity of fire due to water being vacuous. (According to modern Western medicine,) this is an autoimmune dysfunction. Exposure to sunlight may either induce or aggravate this condition.

Diagnosis: The skin lesions are pleomorphic, changeable, and come and go. Frequently there is erythema accompanied by slight edema. The erythema is distributed in a typical butterfly pattern on the face. There may also be hemorrhagic erythema on the ends of the extremities. Common systemic signs and symptoms include fever, arthralgia, malaise and general lassitude. Sometimes the heart may be involved in which case there may be impairment of the cardiac muscles, hypercardia, pleurisy, interstitial pneumonia, nephritis, digestive tract bleeding, and enlargement of the liver and spleen as well as psychopathy and sudden loss of consciousness. Laboratory findings reveal normal pigmented anemia of the medium type, decrease in both leukocytes and thrombocytes, acceleration of blood sedimentation, presence of "lupus" cells in the peripheral blood or bone marrow, lowered levels of serum albumin and increase of globulin, and the presence of erythrocytes and protein in the urine. Accompanying symptoms are lumbar soreness, limpness of the limbs, tinnitus, loss of hair, heat in the five hearts, night sweats, constipation, scant, red urine, and abnormal menstruation in females. The tongue is red and fissured and the pulse is thready and rapid, all of which indicate yin vacuity.

Treatment

Internal Medication:

In order to nourish yin, clear heat, and cool the blood, use Radix Scrophulariae Ningpoensis (*Xuan Shen*), Radix Rehmanniae (*Sheng Di*), Tuber Ophiopogonis Japonicae (*Mai Dong*), Fructus Ligustri Lucidi (*Nu Zhen Zi*), Radix Lithospermi Seu Arnebiae (*Hong Tiao Zi Cao*), Radix Glycyrrhizae (*Gan Cao*), and Herba Ecliptae Prostratae (*Han Lian Cao*), 15g @. Decoct with water and take. If accompanied by menstrual irregularity, add Radix Angelicae Sinensis (*Dang Gui*) and Radix Albus Paeoniae Lactiflorae (*Bai Shao*), 15g @. In case of albuminuria, add Herba Capsellae Bursa-pastoris (*Ji Cai*), 30g. For soreness and pain of the lumbus and waist, add Radix Dipsaci (*Xu Duan*) and Cortex Eucommiae Ulmoidis (*Du Zhong*), 15g @. For night sweats, and spontaneous sweating, add raw Concha Ostreae (*Sheng Mu Li*) and Fructus Levis Tritici (*Fu Xiao Mai*), 30g @.

External Therapies:

1) Apply a 20% solution of Radix Glycyrrhizae (*Gan Cao*).

2) *Qing Dai Gao* (20) may be used externally.

2. Chronic Disciform Lupus Erythematosus
Mai Xing Pan Zhuang Hong Ban Xing Lang Chuang

Pathogenesis and pathophysiology: Same as for systemic lupus erythematosus.

Diagnosis: The lesions consist of erythema with a distinct border and an atrophic, depressed center. These are accompanied by telangiectasis and adhesive scaling. The distribution of these lesions is more or less symmetrical. The labial mucosa may exhibit grayish white ulcerations with shallow festering. The progress of this disease is slow with no systemic symptoms. Only a few exceptional cases will evolve into systemic erythema causing other pathological conditions within the body.

Treatment

Internal Medication:

In order to nourish yin and supplement the kidneys, administer *Liu Wei Di Huang Wan* (46), 15g per time, 2 times per day.

External Therapies:

Same as for systemic lupus.

3. Dermatomyositis
Pi Ji Yan

Pathogenesis and pathophysiology: This condition is caused by stasis and stagnation of the qi and blood (due to general weakness of the health) which obstruct the channels and connecting vessels.

Diagnosis: Skin conditions include substantial facial edema, especially of the eyelids, with no remarkable depression upon pressure but followed by light purple erythema. There may also be symmetrical puffy erythema on the interior aspect of the limbs and on the neck, chest and shoulder. Muscular conditions primarily involve the striated muscles of which the proximal muscles of the four extremities and of the pharynx are most likely to be affected. There may be such symptoms as weakness of the muscles, locomotive impairment, difficulty walking and swallowing, and change in voice. Redness and swelling of the muscles may occur in a few cases, in which case there are also tender spots and pain of the affected muscles. Other symptoms include irregular fever and arthralgia. About 20-30% of cases are complicated by internal malignant tumors. Creatine levels in the urine over a 24 hour period may be as remarkably high as 200-1000 milligrams or higher. Pathological examination of the muscles may also be of diagnostic value.

Treatment

Internal Medication:

In order to boost the qi, activate the blood, and open the connecting vessels, use Radix Astragali Membranacei (*Huang Qi*) and Radix Codonopsis Pilosulae (*Dang Shen*), 25g @, Radix Angelicae Sinensis (*Dang Gui*), Rhizoma Atractylodis Macrocephalae (*Bai Zhu*), Cortex Eucommiae Ulmoidis (*Du Zhong*), Radix Glycyrrhizae (*Gan Cao*), Radix Salviae Miltiorrhizae (*Dan Shen*), and Caulis Milletiae Seu Spatholobi (*Ji Xue Teng*), 15g @, and Flos Carthami Tinctorii (*Hong Hua*), Lumbricus (*Di Long*), and Radix Achyranthis Bidentatae (*Niu Xi*), 10g @. Decoct with water and take.

External Therapies:

1) Acupuncture: *Qu Chi* (LI 11), *He Gu* (LI 4), *Nei Guan* (Per 6), *Wai Guan* (TH 5), *Jian Yu* (LI 15), and *Jian Jing* (GB 21) for the upper limbs and *Huan Tiao* (GB 30), *Feng Shi* (GB 31), *Fu Tu* (ST 32), *Xue Hai* (SP 10), *Zu San Li* (ST 36), and *Yang Ling Quan* (GB 34) for lower limbs.

2) Appropriate massage (is recommended) to prevent muscular atrophy.

4. Scleroderma
   Ying Pi Bing

Pathogenesis and pathophysiology: This condition is caused by insufficiency of kidney yang and lack of consolidation of the *wei* qi which thus invites attack by external wind and cold pathogens. (As a result,) the skin and muscles are occluded by the pathogens which thus leads to obstruction and disharmony of the *wei* and *ying*.

Diagnosis: This condition is most commonly encountered amongst females. It may be of two types, localized or effusive.

Localized type:

1) Plaque-like lesions of different sizes: The skin may appear tense and waxy with variably tinged plaques. Telangiectasis is also present which tends to occur around the head and facial areas. Depressed, irregular stripes may commonly develop on the scalp.

2) Girdle-like lesions: These tend to be distributed over the limbs and costal areas like a girdle. (The lesions themselves) are similar to the plaque-like areas in terms of shiny skin and pigmentation in the affected area.

3) Guttate lesions: These are whitish or ivory colored, small plaques with a distinctive border and widely spread distribution. They are smooth and shiny with purple-red borders. They feel hard and tend to develop over the body trunk.

Effusive type:

1) The initial symptom is substantial edema. (Following this) the skin gradually hardens and turns waxy bright. There may be increase or depletion of pigment and the hair may fall. The subcutaneous tissues and appendages of the skin are so severely atrophic that they are tightly attached to the bones forming a plaque as hard as a board. Such lesions may be confined to the limbs initially, but later on, they may spread widely.

2) There may be such systemic symptoms as vasomotor disturbances, soreness and pain of the joints, fever, poor appetite, malaise, and

119

emaciation.

3) The digestive tract and the heart and lungs may also be involved.

4) This condition is often accompanied by soreness of the lumbar region, hair loss, loose teeth, aversion to cold, cold limbs, spontaneous sweating, loose stools, impeded sexual function, irregular menstruation, a thready, slow pulse, and a pale, tender tongue, all of which indicate yang vacuity of the kidneys.

Treatment

Internal Medication:

In order to reinforce the yang and scatter cold, regulate the *ying* and *wei* and open the striae of the muscles and skin, modified *Yang He Tang* (5) is prescribed.

External Therapies:

Hong Ling Jiu (24) may be applied as a lotion.

5. Panniculitis
Zhi Mo Yan

Pathogenesis and pathophysiology: This condition is similar to what is called *gua teng chan* (entangled melon vine in TCM). It is caused by destruction of the channels and connecting vessels by damp heat pathogens which (in turn) produce heat and stasis from stagnation and accumulation.

Diagnosis:

1) Fever may be either continuous or there may be remittent high fever. However, two thirds of cases present with recurrent fever which varies in duration from several days to weeks.

2) Subcutaneous nodulation appears in all cases. They may appear at indeterminate times. They are painful locally or upon pressure. They may be followed by mild edema of the surrounding tissues. The nodes feel slightly hard and protrude above the surface of the skin. They are pink or purplish red in color. Occasionally, red plaques may also be noted. Squamous scaling or scabs may sometimes form on the surface of the nodes. The nodes seldom rupture. Once the nodes do become perforated, they become productive and discharge a yellowish, greasy fluid. The number and size of the nodes may vary from several to a dozen and from 0.2 to 10 *cun* with most being 1-3 *cun* (in diameter). They tend to develop around the four extremities and especially on the lower extremities, or the face and cheeks, and on the body trunk.

3) Swelling and pain of the lymph nodes are commonly found in the cervical, supraclavicular, submaxillary, subauditory, and inguinal areas.

4) Other symptoms may include headache, nausea, myalgia, arthralgia, and stomatitis.

5) Histopathological examination is of value.

Treatment

Internal Medication:

In order to activate the blood, remove stasis and obstruction from the connecting vessels, clear heat, and eliminate dampness, administer *Bu Yang Huan Wu Tang* (15) plus Fructus Forsythiae Suspensae (*Lian Qiao*) and Fructus Chaenomelis Lagenariae (*Mu Gua*), 15g @, and Semen Arecae Catechu (*Bing Lang*) and Rhizoma Cyperi Rotundi (*Xiang Fu*), 9g @. Decoct with water and take. (Or use) Squama Manitis Pentadactylis (*Chuan Shan Jia*), Lumbricus (*Di Long*), Sanguis Draconis (*Xue Jie*), and Radix Saussureae Seu Vladimiriae (*Mu Xiang*), 5g @, plus Scolopendra (*Wu Gong*) 1pc. Grind (these) into a fine powder and take (orally) one third of this amount 1 time per day with water. The above mentioned two prescriptions can be used alternately.

External Therapies:

Jin Huang San (18) may be applied externally after mixing with water.

Fifteen

Dyschromatic Skin Diseases

1. Vitiligo
Bai Dian Feng

Pathogenesis and pathophysiology: This is called *bai bo feng* (adverse white wind) in the classics. It is believed to be caused by the invasion of the skin by wind and dampness. (According to modern Western medicine,) it is due to a dysfunction in the metabolism of tyrosinase into dihydroxyphenylalanine within the melanocytes. (As a result,) melanin cannot be produced. Mental disturbance, nervous dysfunction, and disorders of the endocrine system often induce this condition.

Diagnosis: Disappearance of the pigment over the affected area gives rise to whitish skin with a distinctive border. Hair in affected areas likewise turns white as well. Pigmentation, distributed either symmetrically or irregularly around the border of the areas, may be present. Sensitivity of and secretions in the affected areas are normal. There are typically no subjective symptoms.

Treatment

Internal Medication:

In order to dispel wind and eliminate dampness use :

1) *Bai Bo Pian:* Radix Lithospermi Seu Arnebiae (*Hong Tiao Zi Cao*), Lignum Dalbergiae Odoriferae (*Chen Zhen Xiang*), Rhizoma Paridis (*Zhong Leng*), Rhizoma Stephaniae Cepharanthae (*Bai Yao*

123

Zi), Radix Cynanchi Atrati (*Bai Wei*), Rhizoma Atractylodis (*Cang Zhu*), Flos Carthami Tinctorii (*Hong Hua*), Semen Pruni Persicae (*Tao Ren*), and raw Radix Polygoni Multiflori (*He Shou Wu*), 50g @, Os Sepiae Seu Sepiellae (*Wu Zei Gu*) and Radix Glycyrrhizae (*Gan Cao*), 35g @, Radix Gentianae Scabrae (*Long Dan Cao*), 20g, and Fructus Tribuli Terrestris (*Bai Ji Li*), 750g. Grind (the above) into a fine powder and make into tablets each weighing 1 gram. Take 10g each time, 2 times per day.

2) Take Fructus Tribuli Terrestris (*Bai Ji Li*), 6g each time, 2 times per day.

3) Take *Xi Xian Wan*, which consists of an unspecified amount of Herba Siegesbeckiae (*Xi Jian Cao*). This ingredient should be mixed with rice wine (*Huang Jiu*) and then steamed and dried in the sun 9 times before being ground into powder. Pill with honey into the size of Chinese parasol tree seeds (approximately the size of a pea).

4) Take equal parts powdered Periostracum Cicadae (*Chan Tui*) and Herba Menthae (*Bo He*), 2g each time, 2 times per day.

External Therapies:

1) A 30% tincture of Fructus Psoraleae Corylifoliae (*Bu Gu Zhi*) may be used externally.

2) Powder equal parts Rhizoma Typhonii (*Bai Fu Zi*) and Sulphur (*Liu Huang*), mix with ginger juice, and apply externally.

2. Freckles
Que Ban

Pathogenesis and pathophysiology: The root cause of this condition is stagnation of fire in the blood phase of the *sun luo* (minor, superficial capillaries) aggravated by external attack of wind pathogens. It is also related to heredity.

Diagnosis: Freckles are brownish, yellowish, or dark brown spots which vary from the size of a pinhead to a hyacinth bean and have a distinct border. In most cases, they are either densely (clustered) or scattered. They tend to develop around the face, sides of the neck, and on the dorsal aspects of the hands. They may also extend symmetrically to the chest and abdomen and to the interior aspects of the four extremities. (This condition) is often more pronounced during the summer while in the fall and winter the pigmentation may fade a bit.

Treatment

1) Grind Rhizoma Typhonii (*Bai Fu Zi*), Radix Angelicae (*Bai Zhi*), and Talcum (*Hua Shi*), 6g @, and Semen Phaseoli Munginis (*Lu Dou*), 250g, and mix thoroughly. Rub the affected area (with this powder) in the morning and evenings after having washed the face.

2) Grind Bombyx Batryticatus (*Jiang Can*), Semen Pharbitidis (*Qian Niu Zi*), and Herba Cum Radice Asari Seiboldi (*Xi Xin*), 60g @, into a fine powder and pill with honey into the size of marbles. Apply the herbs externally when washing the face 2 times per day.

3. Skin Melanosis
Pi Fu Hei Bian Bing

Pathogenesis and pathophysiology: This is called *li hei* (dark appearance) in the classics and is due to exhaustion of kidney yin. (According to modern Western medicine,) because this is a kind of photodermatitis, this condition may be due to either deficiency of vitamin B or to chronic poisoning due to longterm contact with coal-tar products.

125

Diagnosis: This skin condition tends to focus on the face and neck. Occasionally it appears on the forearm, the dorsal aspect of the hands, and on the chest. The skin may look red at first after exposure to the sun. Later, punctate and reticular dark brown plaques may follow. There are no subjective symptoms.

Treatment

Internal Medication:

In order to nourish yin and supplement the kidneys, administer modified *Liu Wei Di Huang Tang* which consists of Radix Coquitus Rehmanniae (*Shu Di*), 30g, Fructus Lycii Chinensis (*Gou Qi Zi*), and Radix Dioscoreae Oppositae (*Shan Yao*), 15g @, Radix Morindae Officinalis (*Ba Ji Tian*), Herba Epimedii (*Xian Ling Pi*), Fructus Corni Officinalis (*Shan Zhu Yu*), Sclerotium Poriae Cocoris (*Fu Ling*), and Rhizoma Alismatis (*Ze Xie*), 12g @. Decoct with water and take.

External Therapies:

1) Treat the same way as for freckles.

2) Tincture Rhizoma Atractylodis Macrocephalae (*Bai Zhu*) in 120ml of white vinegar. Soak for three days. Then apply externally.

4. Macula Lutea
Huang E Ban

Pathogenesis and pathophysiology: This condition develops as a result of spleen vacuity complicated by wind pathogens. (According to modern Western medicine,) most cases are associated with exposure to sunshine and fluctuations in endocrine hormones after conception. A few cases are related to certain chronic diseases, such as liver disease, tuberculosis, and neoplasms of the internal organs.

Diagnosis: The lesions are distributed symmetrically over the face, in the vicinity of the ocular fossa, and around the forehead, cheeks, nose and mouth. They may appear light brownish and sometimes look like the wings of a butterfly. There are no subjective symptoms.

Treatment

Internal Medication:

In order to dispel wind and strengthen the spleen, administer Radix Astragali Membranacei (*Huang Qi*) and Radix Rehmanniae (*Sheng Di*), 15g @, Fructus Tribuli Terrestris (*Bai Ji Li*) and Rhizoma Atractylodis Macrocephalae (*Bai zhu*), 9g @, Herba Spirodelae Seu Lemnae (*Fu Ping*) and Radix Rubrus Paeoniae Lactiflorae (*Chi Shao*), 6g @, and Periostracum Cicadae (*Chan Tui*), 3g. Decoct with water and take.

External Therapies:

Use the same therapy as for freckles.

Sixteen

Disorders of the Skin Appendages

1. Seborrheic Dermatitis
Zhi Yi Xing Pi Yan

Pathogenesis and pathophysiology: The condition results from dryness due to long-standing stagnation after invasion by wind evil. In the classics, the squamous type is called *bai xie feng* (white clipping dermatitis) and the scabious type is called *mian you feng* (face wandering dermatitis). (According to modern Western medicine,) this condition is caused by hypersecretion of the sebaceous glands and scratching which leads to secondary infection. *The Golden Mirror of Ancestral Medicine* states: "*Bai xie feng* first develops in the scalp and then extends to the face, ears, and neck, causing dryness and itching. If the condition persists, it produces white clippings (dandruff)." Again, "*Mian you feng* ... develops on the face. At first, the face and eyes are puffy. Itching is felt as if insects were crawling on the skin. White clippings on the dry skin are frequently observed. The subsequent symptoms are extreme itching which one cannot refrain from scratching which is then productive of a yellowish, serous fluid in cases predominated by damp heat and bloody serous fluid in cases predominantly by wind dryness."

Diagnosis: Young adults are most likely to be affected. Infants are the second largest group (as in cradle cap). This condition frequently focuses on those areas densely supplied with sebaceous glands, such as the scalp, face (especially the eyebrow arch and both sides of the nose), external auditory meatus, axillae, upper chest, and the back. It is also noted that the condition spreads down from the head. Lesions may consist of red or pink macules tinged with a light yellow color and characterized by variable size, distinct borders, and irregular margins. In the squamous type, the lesions look like flakes with greasy clippings on the surface which may fall off in considerable amounts when combing. In the scabious type, scabs may form on a base of thickening and accumulation of greasy clippings. Ulcers productive of serous fluid may result from scratching due to itching.

Treatment

Internal Medication:

For the scabious type, in order to primarily clear heat and eliminate dampness, use *Wu Wei Xiao Du Yin* (12) plus Herba Artemesiae Capillaris (*Yin Chen Hao*), 15g, and Fructus Gardeniae Jasminoidis (*Zhi Zi*) and Radix Et Rhizoma Rhei (*Da Huang*), 3g @. Decoct with water and take.

For the squamous type, in order to clear heat and cool the blood, nourish the blood and moisten dryness, administer Radix Polygoni Multiflori (*He Shou Wu*), Radix Rehmanniae (*Sheng Di*), and Herba Ecliptae Prostratae (*Han Lian Cao*), 15g @, and Cortex Radicis Moutan (*Mu Dan Pi*), Radix Angelicae Sinensis (*Dang Gui*), Radix Rubrus Paeoniae Lactiflorae (*Chi Shao*), and Fructus Ligustri Lucidi (*Nu Zhen Zi*), 10g @.

External Therapies:

1) *Bai Xie Feng Ding* (23) may be used externally.

2) *Run Ji Gao* (22) may be used externally.

3) Wash with a decoction of Cortex Radicis Dictamni (*Bai Xian Pi*), Radix Sophorae Flavescentis (*Ku Shen*), Flos Chrysanthemi Indici (*Ye Ju Hua*), Radix Et Rhizoma Rhei (*Da Huang*) and Herba Senecionis Scandentis (*Qian Li Guang*), 30g @.

4) Apply externally of 5% sulphur ointment.

2. Common Acne
Xun Chang Cuo Chuang

Pathogenesis and pathophysiology: The ancient name for this condition is *fei feng fen chi* (acne due to lung wind) which is caused by accumulation of heat in the three channels of the lungs, spleen, and stomach. (According to modern Western medicine,) the maturing sex glands during puberty enhance the secretion of the endocrine system thus leading to hypersteatosis and occlusion of the sebaceous glands associated with the hair follicles. Chronic suppurative folliculitis is the subsequent result when complicated by secondary bacterial infection. Overeating fats and carbohydrates and indigestion are often (also) precipitating factors.

Diagnosis: Acne tends to develop around the areas densely supplied with sebaceous glands, such as the face, upper chest, and back. Lesions are often multiform. Comedones are typically the earliest sign. Papules, suppuration, nodulation, abscess, and scarring occur sequentially in the course of development. At the early stage, one can express the comedones and squeeze out a tiny blackhead the size of millet with some yellow white substance.

Treatment

Internal Medication:

In order to clear lung and stomach heat and to disinhibit lung qi, (one can use either):

1) *Pei Pa Qing Fei Yin:* Folium Eriobatryae (*Pei Pa Ye*) and Cortex Radicis Moutan (*Dan Pi*), 15g @, and Radix Codonopsis Pilosulae (*Dang Shen*), Radix Glycyrrhizae (*Gan Cao*), Rhizoma Coptidis Chinensis (*Huang Lian*), and Cortex Phellodendri (*Huang Bai*), 9g @. Decoct with water and take.

2) In chronic tenacious cases, powder equal portions of Radix Salviae Miltiorrhizae (*Dan Shen*), Radix Codonopsis Pilosulae (*Dang Shen*),

131

Radix Sophorae Flavescentis (*Ku Shen*), and Radix Glehniae Littoralis (*Sha Shen*) and mix with mashed Semen Juglandis Regiae (*Hu Tao Ren*). Make into pills the size of Chinese parasol tree seeds. Take 10g with water every night.

External Therapies:

1) *Dian Dao San Xi Ji* (29) may be used externally.

2) *San Huang Xi Ji* (28) may be used as a lotion.

3. Acne Rosacea
Jiu Zha Bi

Pathogenesis and pathophysiology: This condition results from stomach fire accumulating in the lungs with blood stasis congealing and binding. (According to modern Western medicine,) it is caused by long term dilation of the local blood capillaries which is due to dysfunction of the vasomotor nerves. Predilection for alcohol, indigestion, endocrine imbalance, and persistent external climate acting upon the skin, such as working under high temperature, sunburn, and exposure to wind, are all precipitating factors.

Diagnosis: The skin lesion is restricted to the center of the face from the forehead to the chin and especially to the nasal region. The initial symptoms are red spots which occur paroxysmally and transiently which may be followed by groups of papules and suppurative blisters varying in size from pinheads to soybeans. These red spots later will not subside and give rise to dilation of the capillaries. In severe cases the local tissues are found to have thickened and a hammer-nose is (thus) formed. As a rule, there are no subjective symptoms.

Treatment

Internal Medication:

In order to clear heat and cool the blood, to activate the blood and eliminate stasis, decoct and take *Liang Xue Si Wu Tang* (14).

External Therapies:

1) *Dian Dao Xan Xi Ji* (29) may be applied as a lotion.

2) Acne Rosacea Ointment may be used externally: Lithargyrum (*Mi Tuo Seng*), 60g, Radix Scrophulariae Ningpoensis (*Xuan Shen*) and Sulphur (*Liu Huang*), 30g @, and Calomelas (*Qing Fen*), 25g. Grind these into a fine powder and mix with honey into a paste before external application.

4. Body Odor
Chou Han Zheng

Pathogenesis and pathophysiology: Another name for this condition is *ti qi* (body qi). (According to modern Western medicine,) it is a kind of specific bad odor emitted by unsaturated fatty acids generated by bacterial action upon the organic substances excreted by the major sweat glands.

Diagnosis: This condition is common in youths of both sexes but especially among young women. The bad odor arises from those areas supplied by large sweat glands, such as the axillae, nipples, umbilicus, pubis, and perineum.

Treatment

1) Hircus Powder: Lithargyrum (*Mi Tuo Seng*), 12g, *San Xian Dan*[1],

---

[1]   *San Xian Dan* is a ready made patent medicine. According to *Yan Yi Da Quan (The Great Compendium of Ulcerous Medicine)*, it is composed of Mercury (*Shui Yin*), 50g, and Alum (*Ku Fan*) and Niter (*Ya Xiao*), 60g @. "Put the powdered mixture of the above three ingredients in a wok and cover with a porcelain bowl which has been rubbed inside and out with a slice of ginger so as to prevent explosion. Cover the bowl and seal with a paste made of salted earth. Fifteen hundred grams of charcoal is needed (for fuel. This charcoal

and Calomelas (*Qing Fen*), 9g @, and powdered Talcum (*Hua Shi Fen*), 3g. Calomelas should be ground separately before being mixed with the other powders. Dust (the affected areas) twice per day for 3-5 days.

2) Hircus Lotion: Lithargyrum (*Mi Tuo Seng*), 30g, Alumen (*Ming Fan*), 15g, and 40% formalin, 10 ml. Add up to 100 ml water and apply externally.

3) Lithargyrum Powder: Realgar (*Xiong Huang*), 9g, Sulphur (*Liu Huang*) and Fructus Cnidii Monnieri (*She Chuang Zi*), 6g @, Lithargyrum (*Mi Tuo Seng*), 3g, and Calomelas (*Qing Fen*), 1.5g. Grind into a fine powder for dusting.

5. Alopecia Areata
Ban Tu

Pathogenesis and pathophysiology: This condition is also called *you feng* (greasy wind) in the classics. It is caused by blood vacuity and wind dryness due to insufficiency of kidney yin. (According to modern Western medicine,) mental distress, endocrine impairment, and acute infectious diseases often are precipitating factors. *The Orthodox Manual of Wai Ke* states, "*You feng* is due to blood vacuity which results in the failure to nourish the skin by the ascending qi. The condition is characterized by brightness of the scalp due to emptiness of the hair roots which leads to the hair falling out in patches."

Diagnosis: (This condition manifests as) the sudden appearance of circular or oval patches of baldness without redness, swelling,

---

should surround the entire wok). If the salted earth becomes cracked the fissures should be filled with more salted earth. The duration of processing is about the length of time required to burn three incense sticks. Break the seal and scrape the minerals off the bowl. Grind them into a fine powder and keep them in a porcelain container for use." (Quoted from *Zhong Yao Da Ci Dian* [*Encyclopedia Materia Medica Sinensis*], page 451.)

squamous scaling, or any subjective symptoms. Sometimes, sparse, grayish white hair may grow but which may fall out immediately. Few cases are so severe that there is complete balding, even including the eyebrows, axillary hair, and pubic hair.

Treatment

Internal Medication:

In order to nourish the blood, dispel wind, and supplement the kidneys, *Shen Ying Yang Zhen Dan* is indicated. Take equal portions of Rhizoma Seu Radix Notoptergii (*Qiang Huo*), Fructus Chaenomelis Lagenariae (*Mu Gua*), Rhizoma Gastrodiae Elatae (*Tian Ma*), Radix Albus Paeoniae Lactiflorae (*Bai Shao*), Radix Angelicae Sinensis (*Dang Gui*), Semen Cuscutae (*Tu Si Zi*), Radix Coquitus Rehmanniae (*Shu Di*), and Radix Ligustici Wallichii (*Chuan Xiong*) and grind them into a fine powder. Mix with honey to make pills the size of Chinese parasol tree seeds. Take 10g each time, twice per day with a light salt solution.

External Therapies:

1) Prick the affected area with a plum blossom needle.

2) Apply externally a 25% tincture of Fructus Zanthoxyli Bungeani (*Chuan Jiao*).

3) Mix powdered Radix Aconiti (*Chuan Wu*) with vinegar and apply externally.

Seventeen _____

Congenital & Keratosing Dermatoses

1. Ichthyosis
Yu Lin Bin

Pathogenesis and pathophysiology: Another name for this condition is *she pi xian* (snake skin tinea). It is caused by *ying* and blood insufficiency. (Because) the blood is vacuous, wind is generated. Excessive wind (leads to) blood dryness and thus the skin loses its nourishment. Heredity is an important factor since quite a number of patients' (families) have been afflicted over generations.

Diagnosis: This condition may develop during early childhood. It is aggravated during the winter and subsides in summer. The lesions focus mostly on the exterior aspects of the four limbs and back. In severe cases, they may spread over the entire body. Dryness of the skin is its main characteristic. Brown or dark, fishlike scaling may be noticed on the surface. There are no subjective symptoms.

Treatment

Internal Medication:

In order to nourish the blood, dispel wind, and moisten dryness, administer either *Jia Jian Gui Zhi Dang Gui Tang* (1) or *Run Fu Tang* (11).

External Therapies:

1) Apply externally *Run Ji Gao* (22)

137

2) Mash together Semen Pruni Armeniacae (*Xing Ren*), 30g, and lard (*Zhu You*), 60g, and apply externally.

3) *Gan Cao You* (27) may be used externally.

2. Perifollicular Keratosis
Mao Nong Zhou Wei Jiao Hua Bin

Pathogenesis and pathophysiology: This condition is due to damage and injury of lung and stomach yin by dry qi.

Diagnosis: This condition is common in youths and in the winter. The lesions tend to occur around the lateral aspects of the thighs, the exterior aspect of the forearm, and on the back. (They are characterized by) pinhead- sized, scattered, follicular papules which feel rough like chicken skin. There are no subjective symptoms in most cases.

Treatment

Internal Medication:

In order to clear and nourish the lungs and stomach, decoct with water and take *Sha Shen Mai Dong Tang*: Radix Glehniae Littoralis (*Sha Shen*), Rhizoma Polygonati Odorati (*Yu Zhu*), Semen Dolichoris Lablabis (*Bian Dou*), and Radix Trichosanthis Kirlowii (*Hua Fen*), 9g @, and Radix Glycyrrhizae (*Gan Cao*), 3g.

External Therapies:

1) *Pi Zhi Gao* (40) may be used externally.

2) *Run Ji Gao* (22) may be used externally.

3. Progressive Keratoderma of the Metacarpophalangeal Joints
Jing Xing Zhi Zhang Jiao Pi Zheng

Pathogenesis and pathophysiology: (According to modern Western medicine,) change of sex hormones is presumed related to this condition. (According to TCM,) imbalance of the *chong* and *ren* is the major pathogenic factor. Contact with soap and water often makes this condition worse.

Diagnosis: This condition is common in post-pubescent women from sixteen to thirty years of age. At first, the last section of the thumb, index, and middle fingers of the right hand are noted to be dry, rough, and have less perspiration. Later, the lesions may extend to the other fingers and the palm. In severe cases, patches of scaling may fall off and the local skin looks light reddish or purplish. Sometimes hypertrophy of the corneal layer prohibit the fingers from (normal) movement. Deep fissures are also noted in the area of the skin creases. There is severe pain, (therefore,) when using the fingers. (As a rule,) there are neither ulcerous lesions nor itching. The left hand may also be similarly affected. (But) the dorsal aspect of the hand and forearms are scarcely ever affected.

Treatment

Internal Medication:

In order to supplement the kidneys and enrich yin, take *Liu Wei Di Huang Wan* (46) twice per day, 15g each time.

External Therapies:

1) Wash with a warm, medicinal soup made from Cortex Radicis Lycii (*Di Gu Pi*), Cacumen Biotae Orientalis (*Ce Bai Ye*), Alum (*Ku Fan*), Cortex Phellodendri (*Huang Bai*), and Radix Glycyrrhizae (*Gan Cao*), 30g @.

2) Apply externally either *Gan Cao You* (27) or *Run Ji Gao* (22).

Eighteen

Skin Tumors

1. Keloids
Ba Hen Ge Da

Pathogenesis and pathophysiology: This condition is not actually a skin tumor but is a kind of vegetation of the connective tissue of the skin. Most lesions occur on scars wrought by external wounds, burns, infections, and surgery. Primary cases are also possible.

Diagnosis: Being hairless, the scar is raised above the skin. It is pink or dark red, smooth, and shiny. Capillary dilation is often noted. Keloids feels hard and substantial and vary in size and shape. Pain or itching may often be felt subjectively.

Treatment

1) *Hei Ba Gao*: Black vinegar (*Hei Cu*), 250 ml, Galla Rhi Chinensis (*Wu Bei Zi*), 85g, Scolopendra (*Wu Gong*), 1 piece, and honey (*Feng Mi*), 18g. Grind the herbs and make into a paste before external application.

2) *Ku Shen Zi Gao*: Grind Semen Sophorae Flavescentis (*Ku Shen Zi Fen*), 90g, into a fine powder and mix into a paste with petroleum jelly, 210g. Apply externally after thorough mixing.

2. Basal Cell Carcinoma
Ji Di Xi Bao Ai

Pathogenesis and pathophysiology: This disease is caused by evil qi invading the surface. There it depresses the flesh and skin. Binding and accumulation transform into toxins which flourish.

Diagnosis: Most patients are middle aged. The lesions tend to occur around the head and face. The initial symptom is a waxy nodulation. Dilation of a number of capillary vessels can be observed on its surface. The nodulation grows and expands gradually until a flat center and ulcerative depression is formed. Without a raised border, the irregularly shaped, ulcerous surface may bleed easily. The malignancy of this condition is low. Its course of development is slow during which the tumor simply expands into neighboring areas and invades underlying tissues. Metastasis is unusual.

Treatment

Internal Medication:

In order to scatter nodulation, soften the hard, and resolve toxins, administer *Ju Zhao Wan*: Flos Lonicerae Japonicae (*Jin Yin Hua*), Radix Rhapontici Seu Echinposis (*Lou Lu*), Semen Iridis Pallidae (*Ma Lin Zi*), Semen Strychnotis (*Ma Qian Zi*), and Bulbus Cremastrae (*Shan Ci Gu*), 300g @, Herba Sargassi (*Hai Zao*), Flos Chrysanthemi Morifolii (*Ju Hua*), Rhizoma Sparganii (*San Leng*), and Radix Paridis Polyphyllae (*Zao Xiu*), 200g @, Radix Polygoni Multiflori (*He Shou Wu*), 400g, Scolopendra (*Wu Gong*), 100g, and Rhizoma Coptidis Chinensis (*Huang Lian*), 50g. Grind the (above) herbs into a fine powder. Add water and pill the size of mung beans. Take 3-5 grams each time, 3 times per day.

External Therapies:

1) *Wu Hu Dan* (Five Tiger Elixir): Hydrargyrum (*Shui Yin*), Alumen (*Bai Fan*), Melanteritum (*Qing Fan*), and crystallized Niter (*Ya Xiao*), 180g @ and table salt (*Shi Yen*) 90g. Grind in a mortar until the Hydrargyrum can no longer be seen. The powdered ingredients should be placed in a crucible and heated in order to evaporate the

water. *Dan Tai* (embryonic elixir) is (thus) formed. Seal the lid of the crucible with Gypsum Fibrosum (*Shi Gao*) mixed with salt solution and place the crucible upside down inside a porcelain jar. The lid of the jar should be filled with water taken from lotus leaves, while the interior of the jar should contain 10k of water. The jar should be baked with ignited charcoal heaped over it for two hours. Obtain the elixir after the porcelain jar has cooled. The whitish crystalline elixir is considered the best. Grind these into a fine powder and spread this locally over the affected area or make a paste with the juice strained from cooked rice. Apply to the lesion and bandage.

2) *Chuan Shu Yuan Gao*; Dissolve Venenum Bufonis (*Chan Su*), 10g, in distilled water, 30g. Then add petroleum jelly, 40g, and mix thoroughly before applying externally.

3) Mix equal parts powdered raw Radix Aconiti (*Chuan Wu*) with white vinegar (*Bai Cu*) and honey. Mix thoroughly before applying externally. Change the dressing daily.

Nineteen _____

Occupational Dermatitis

1. Ulcerous Rice-field Immersion Dermatitis
Jin Ji Mi Lan Xing Dao Tian Pi Yan

Pathogenesis and pathophysiology: Called *shui ji chuang* (water immersion lesion), it is caused by the external invasion of water dampness which later turns into heat. (According to modern Western medicine,) this condition results from irritation of the skin by organic substances contained in the water, immersion in water and mud, and from mechanical friction. The higher the water temperature, the higher the incidence.

Diagnosis: This condition appears 1—3 days after working in a rice field. It tends to concentrate on the creases of the fingers or the webs of the toes. The first symptom is itching which is then followed by puffy skin and a whitish appearance due to immersion. Ulceration due to scratching will be productive of serous fluid.

Treatment

Internal Medication:

In order to clear heat and eliminate dampness, administer Flos Lonicerae Japonicae (*Jin Yin Hua*) and Herba Violae Yedoensis (*Zi Hua Di Ding*), 15g @, and Fructus Forsythiae Suspensae (*Lian Qiao*), Radix Rubrus Paeoniae Lactiflorae (*Chi Shao*), Cortex Radicis Moutan (*Dan Pi*), Fructus Gardeniae Jasminoidis (*Zhi Zi*), Rhizoma Atractylodis (*Cang Zhu*), Cortex Phellodendri (*Huang Bai*), Semen Plantaginis (*Che Qian Zi*), and Radix Glycyrrhizae (*Gan Cao*), 9g @.

Decoct with water and take.

External Therapies:

1) *Ku Fan Feng*: Borneolum Syntheticum (*Bing Pian*), 1g, Alum (*Ku Fan*), 25g, zinc oxide, 20g. Add powdered Talcum (*Hua Shi Fen*), until the amount reaches 100g. Dust the mixture over the affected area.

2) *Han Lian Cao Yuan*; Fresh Herba Ecliptae Prostratae (*Han Lian Cao*), 8K (3K if dry), Alumen (*Ming Fan*), 75g, and some petroleum jelly. First mash the Herba Ecliptae Prostratae to obtain the juice. Decoct to get a condensed soup if dry. Reduce the juice in a wok to 500 ml. Add the Alumen and then add petroleum jelly until the total (weight of the mixture) reaches 1500g. Adding a small amount of Borneol will get better results. (Finally,) add benzoic acid as a preservative. Use as an ointment.

3) Immerse the diseased area in a decoction made from Pericarpium Punicae Ganati (*Shi Liu Pi*).

2. Asphalt Dermatitis
Li Qing Pi Yan

Pathogenesis and pathophysiology: This condition arises as a result of hat produced from asphalt toxins. As a rule, this dermatitis occurs upon contact with asphalt and exposure to sunlight.

Diagnosis: The lesions tend to develop on exposed areas, such as the face, neck, hands, and feet. They may extend over the entire body. Erythema, desquamation, ulceration productive of serous fluid, and acneiform dermatitis (are common). The subjective symptoms are slight itching accompanied by such systemic symptoms as headache, nausea, general lassitude, and high fever.

Treatment

Internal Medication:

In order to cool the blood, clear heat, and resolve toxins, use Radix Rehmanniae (*Sheng Di*), 25g @, Radix Lithospermi Seu Arnebiae (*Hong Tiao Zi Cao*), Flos Lonicerae Japonicae (*Jin Yin Hua*), Herba Violae Yedoensis (*Zi Hua Di Ding*), and Radix Isatidis Seu Baphicacanthi (*Ban Lan Gen*), 15g, and Cortex Radicis Moutan (*Dan Pi*), Radix Rubrus Paeoniae Lactiflorae (*Chi Shao*), Radix Scutellariae Baicalensis (*Huang Qin*), Fructus Gardeniae Jasminoidis (*Zhi Zi*), Radix Glycyrrhizae (*Gan Cao*), and prepared Radix Et Rhizoma Rhei (*Zhi Da Huang*), 10g @. Decoct with water and take. In case of ulceration and production of serous fluid, add Herba Phyllanthi Urinariae (*Zhen Zhu Cao*), 30g, and Semen Plantaginis (*Che Qian Zi*), 15g.

External Therapies:

Apply *Qing Dai Gao* (20) in case of absence of ulceration and serous fluid generation. Cold compresses made from a decoction of Cortex Phellodendri (*Huang Bai*) and Radix Glycyrrhizae (*Gan Cao*), 50g @, are recommended.

3. Erythema due to Irritation by Fire
Huo Ji Hong Ban

Pathogenesis and pathophysiology: This is called *huo bang chuang* (fire mark lesion) in the classics. (According to modern Western medicine,) it results from reticular erythema and pigmentation due to long-term exposure of the body surface to high temperature. Most victims are boilermen, heat-treatment, and forge workers.

Diagnosis: Congested skin leads to reticular erythema, which turns from an original light pink to purple brown until at last reticular symptoms except for a burning sensation in severe cases.

Treatment

1) Apply cold compresses made from a decoction of Radix Glycyr-rhizae (*Gan Cao*), 60g.

2) *San Huang Xi Ji* (28) may be used externally.

4. Vegetable Farmer's Dermatitis
Cai Nong Pi Yan

Pathogenesis and pathophysiology: During the height of vegetable production, such a condition may develop due to longterm contact with soil and immersion (in water).

Diagnosis: Skin lesions are mainly located on the soles, sides of the feet, and bends of the toes. The heels and ankles may also be involved in severe cases. The basic lesion is whitish in appearance due to immersion. In severe cases, ulceration is common and is followed by papular or pustular conditions. The patient feels pain and itching subjectively.

Treatment

1) Same as for (the treatment) of ulcerative rice-field immersion dermatitis.

2) Wash (the affected area) with a decoction made of Radix Cynanchi Panniculati (*Xu Chang Xing*), 100g.

3) In cases complicated by infection, take internally a decoction of Radix Cynanchi Panniculati (*Xu Chang Xing*), Rhizoma Smilacis Glabrae (*Tu Fu Ling*), and Flos Lonicerae Japonicae (*Jin Yin Hua*), 30g @. Decoct with water and take.

Appendix I: Prescriptions

(1) Jia Jian Gui Zhi Dang Gui Tang: Rhizoma Polygonati Odorati (*Yu Zhu*) and Semen Sesami Indici (*Hei Ma Zhi*), 15g @, Radix Polygoni Multiflori (*He Shou Wu*), Radix Angelicae Sinensis (*Dang Gui*), Radix Albus Paeoniae Lactiflorae (*Bai Shao*), Radix Gentianae Macrophyllae (*Qin Jiao*), and Fructus Zizyphi Jujubae (*Da Zao*), 10g @, Radix Praeparatus Glycyrrhizae (*Zhi Gan Cao*) and Ramulus Cinnamomi (*Gui Zhi*), 5g @. Decoct with water and take.

Functions and indications: Nourishes the blood and dispels wind in the treatment of ichthyosis and static regressive psoriasis, etc.

(2) Jia Wei Yu Ping Feng San: Radix Astragali Membranacei (*Huang Qi*), Radix Angelicae Sinensis (*Dang Gui*), and Radix Glycyrrhizae (*Gan Cao*), 30g @, Rhizoma Atractylodis Macrocephalae (*Bai Zhu*) and Radix Ledebouriellae Sesloidis (*Fang Feng*), 15g @. Decoct with water and take.

Functions and indications: Consolidates the surface and dispels wind in the treatment of urticaria, etc.

(3) Xiao Feng San: Herba Seu Flos Schizonepetae Tenuifoliae (*Jing Jie Sui*, added to decoction shortly before the end of cooking), Radix Ledebouriellae Sesloidis (*Fang Feng*), Radix Angelicae Sinensis (*Dang Gui*), Radix Sophorae Flavescentis (*Ku Shen*), Rhizoma Atractylodis (*Cang Zhu*), Semen Cannabis Sativae (*Huo Ma Ren*), Fructus Arctii (*Niu Bang Zi*), Rhizoma Anemarrhenae (*Zhi Mu*), Caulis Akebiae Mutong (*Mu Tong*), 10g @, Radix Rehmanniae (*Sheng Di*) and Radix Glycyrrhizae (*Gan Cao*), 5g @, Gypsum Fibrosum (*Shi Gao*), 30g (cook first), and Periostracum Cicadae (*Chan Tui*), 3g. Decoct with water and take.

Functions and indications: Relieves the surface and dispels wind in the treatment of all kinds of acute dermatitis

(4) Dang Gui Si Ni Tang: Radix Angelicae Sinensis (*Dang Gui*), Ramulus Cinnamomi (*Gui Zhi*), Radix Albus Paeoniae Lactiflorae (*Bai Shao*), Caulis Akebiae Mutong (*Mu Tong*), Fructus Zizyphi Jujubae (*Da Zao*), 10g @, Herba Cum Radice Asari Seiboldi (*Xi Xin*), and Radix Praeparatus Glycyrrhizae (*Zhi Gan Cao*), 3g @. Decoct with water and take.

Functions and indications: Warms the channels and scatters cold in the treatment of frostbite, etc.

(5) *Yang He Tang*: Radix Coquitus Rehmanniae (*Shu Di*), 30g, Semen Sinapis Albae (*Bai Jie Zi*) 6g, Herba Ephedrae (*Ma Huang*), Radix Praeparatus Glycyrrhizae (*Zhi Gan Cao*), and Ramulus Cinnamomi (*Gui Zhi*), 3g @, Rhizoma Praeparata Zingiberis (*Pao Jiang*), 1.5g, Colla Cornu Cervi (*Lu Jiao*), 9g (melted separately). Decoct with water and take.

Functions and indications: Assists yang and scatters cold in the treatment of scleroderma

(6) *Qing Hao Yi Ren Tang*: Herba Artemesiae Chinghao (*Qing Hao*), Herba Agastachis Seu Pogostemi (*Huo Xiang*), Herba Eupatorii (*Pei Lan*), Cortex Radicis Lycii (*Di Gu Pi*), and Cortex Phellodendri (*Huang Bai*), 10g @, Folium Isatidis (*Da Qing Ye*), Herba Cum Radice Taraxaci Mongolici (*Pu Gong Ying*), Radix Sophorae Flavescentis (*Ku Shen*), and Flos Lonicerae Japonicae (*Jin Yin Hua*), 15g, raw Semen Coicis Lachryma-jobi (*Sheng Yi Ren*), 30g. Decoct with water and take.

Functions and indications: Eliminates dampness and clears summerheat in the treatment of summertime dermatitis, etc.

(7) *Qing Shu Tang*: Fructus Forsythiae Suspensae (*Lian Qiao*), Radix Trichosanthis Kirlowii (*Hua Fen*), Talcum (*Hua Shi*), and Flos Lonicerae Japonicae (*Jin Yin Hua*), 12g @, Radix Rubrus Paeoniae Lactiflorae (*Chi Shao*), Semen Plantaginis (*Che Qian Zi*), and Rhizoma Alismatis (*Ze Xie*), 9g @, Radix Glycyrrhizae (*Gan Cao*), 3g. Decoct with water and take.

Functions and indications: Dispels toxins and clears summerheat in the treatment of swelling due to furuncles, pyoderma, etc.

(8) *Bi Xie Shen Shi Tang*: Raw Semen Coicis Lachryma-jobi (*Sheng Yi Ren*) and Talcum (*hua Shi*), 30g @, Rhizoma Dioscoreae Hypoglaucae (*Bi Xie*), and Sclerotium Poriae Cocoris (*Fu Ling*), 12g @, Cortex Phellodendri (*Huang Bai*), Cortex Radicis Moutan (*Dan Pi*), and Rhizoma Alismatis (*Ze Xie*), 9g @, Medulla Tetrapanacis Papyriferi (*Tong Cao*), 6g. Decoct with water and take.

Functions and indications: Clears heat and eliminates dampness in the treatment of acute eczema, contact dermatitis, etc.

(9) *Jian Pi Shen Shi Tang*: Radix Codonopsis Pilosulae (*Dang Shen*), Sclerotium Poriae Cocoris (*Fu Ling*), Rhizoma Alismatis (*Ze Xie*), 12g @, Rhizoma Atractylodis Macrocephalae (*Bai Zhu*), and Fructus Zizyphii Jujubae (*Da Zao*), 9g @, Semen Dolichoris Lablabis (*Bai Bian Dou*), and Semen Coicis Lachryma-jobi (*Yi Ren*), 15g @, Radix Dioscoreae Oppositae (*Shan Yao*), 24g, Pericarpium Citri Reticulatae (*Chen Pi*), and Radix Platycodi Grandiflori (*Jie Gen*), 5g @. Decoct with water and take.

Functions and indications: Invigorates the spleen and eliminates dampness in the treatment of infantile eczema with constitutional vacuity, chronic pediatric urticaria, etc.

(10) *Di Huang Yin*: Radix Coquitus Rehmanniae (*Shu Di*), 30g, Radix Rehmanniae (*Sheng Di*), and Rhizoma Polygoni Multiflori (*He Shou Wu*), 15g @, Radix Angelicae Sinensis (*Dang Gui*), Cortex Radicis Moutan (*Dan Pi*), Radix Scrophulariae Ningpoensis (*Yuan Sheng*), and Fructus Tribuli Terrestris (*Bai Ji Li*), 10g @, Bombyx Batryticatus (*Jiang Can*), and Radix Glycyrrhizae (*Gan Cao*), 5g @, and Flos Carthami Tinctorii (*Hong Hua*), 3g. Decoct with water and take.

Functions and indications: Nourishes the blood and moistens dryness in the treatment of chronic eczema, etc.

(11) *Run Fu Tang*: Radix Scrophulariae Ningpoensis (*Yuan Shen*), Tuber Ophiopogonis Japonicae (*Mai Dong*), Ramulus Uncariae Cum Uncis (*Gou Teng*), Radix Rubrus Paeoniae Lactiflorae (*Chi Shao*), Cortex Radicis Moutan (*Dan Pi*), and Cortex Radicis Dictamni (*Bai Xian Pi*), 10g @. Decoct with water and take.

Functions and indications: Generates fluids and moistens dryness in the treatment of pruritus, etc.

(12) *Wu Wei Xiao Du Yin*: Flos Lonicerae Japonicae (*Jin Yin Hua*), Flos Chrysanthemi Indici (*Ye Ju Hua*), Herba Cum Radice Taraxaci Mongolici (*Pu Gong Ying*), Herba Violae Yedoensis (*Zhi Hua Di Ding*), 15g @, Radix Semiaquilegiae (*Qing Tian Kui*), 10g. Decoct with water and take.

Functions and indications: Resolves toxins and precipitates fire in the treatment of pyoderma, swelling due to furuncles (and boils), etc.

(13) *Sheng Di Yin Hua Tang*: Radix Rehmanniae (*Sheng Di*), 30g, Flos Lonicerae Japonicae (*Jin Yin Hua*), 25g, Radix Scrophulariae Ningpoensis (*Yuan Shen*), Herba Violae Yedoensis (*Zi Hua Di Ding*), and Folium Isatidis (*Da Qing Ye*), 15g @, Radix Rubrus Paeoniae Lactiflorae (*Chi Shao*), 10g, Periostracum Cicadae (*Chan Tui*), 3g. Decoct with water and take.

Functions and indications: Cools the blood and precipitates fire in the treatment of lacquer dermatitis, etc.

(14) *Liang Xue Si Wu Tang*: Radix Rehmanniae (*Sheng Di*), 25g, Radix Rubrus Paeoniae Lactiflorae (*Chi Shao*), Radix Angelicae Sinensis (*Dang Gui*), Radix Scutellariae Baicalensis (*Huang Qin*), Sclerotium Poriae Cocoris (*Fu Ling*), and Flos Carthami Tinctorii (*Hong Hua*), 10g @, Radix Ligustici Wallichii (*Chuan Xiong*), Pericarpium Citri Reticulatae (*Chen Pi*), Radix Glycyrrhizae (*Gan Cao*), and Rhizoma Recens Zingiberis (*Sheng Jiang*), 5g @. Decoct with water and take.

Functions and indications: Cools the blood and dispels stasis in the treatment of acne rosacea, etc.

(15) *Bu Yang Huan Wu Tang*: Radix Astragali Membranacei (*Huang Qi*), 15g, Radix Rubrus Paeoniae Lactiflorae (*Chi Shao*), 12g, Lumbricus (*Di Long*), Semen Pruni Persicae (*Tao Ren*), and Flos Carthami Tinctorii (*Hong Hua*), 9g @, Radix Angelicae Sinensis (*Dang Gui*) and Radix Ligustici Wallichii (*Chuan Xiong*), 6g @. Decoct with water and take.

Functions and indications: Activates the blood and dispels stasis in the treatment of panniculitis, etc.

(16) *Qian Chui Gao*: Skinned Semen Ricini Communis (*Bi Ma Zi Rou*), 150g, powdered fresh Colophonium (*Song Xiang*), 300g, Minium (*Qian Dan*), and Cinnabar (*Zhu Sha*), 60g @, Oleum Camelliae (*Cha You*), 50g, and Calomelas (*Qing Fen*), 30g. Mash the Semen Ricini (into a paste) in a stone mortar. Gradually add the powdered Colophonium and mix thoroughly before adding the Calomelas, Cinnabar, and Minium. Oleum Camelliae is added last. Make a paste by pestelling 1000 times. Spread the paste on paper (and allow to dry). (Before applying,) melt (the paste slightly) by steaming.

Functions and indications: Relieves swelling and stops pain, evacuates pus and removes necrotic tissue in the treatment of swelling due to furuncles, perforated furuncles, etc.

(17) *Tai Yi Gao*: Radix Scrophulariae Ningpoensis (*Yuan Shen*), Radix Angelicae (*Bai Zhi*), Radix Angelicae Sinensis (*Dang Gui*), Cortex Cinnamomi (*Rou Gui*), Radix Rubrus Paeoniae Lactiflorae (*Chi Shao*), Radix Et Rhizoma Rhei (*Da Huang*), Radix Rehmanniae (*Sheng Di*), Semen Momordicae Cochinensis (*Mu Bei Zi*), 60g @, Resina Ferulae (*E Wei*), Myrrha (*Mo Yao*), 9g @, Crinis Carbonisatus (*Xue Yu Tan*), 30g, Gummi Olibanum (*Ru Xiang*), 15g, Minium (*Qian Dan*), 1200g, roasted sesame oil (*Xiang You*), 2500g, Ramulus Salicis (*Liu Zhi*), and Ramulus Sophorae Japonicae (*Huai Zhi*), 100 sections @. Fry all the ingredients, except Minium, in roasted sesame oil until they all become desiccated. Add the Minium after removing the dregs. One hundred ninety-five grams of Minium should be added to 500g of oil. The paste is ready when it is thoroughly mixed.

Functions and indications: Disperses swelling and disperses inflammation, resolves toxins and generates (new) tissue in the treatment of swelling due to furuncles, perforated furuncles, etc.

(18) *Jin Huang San*: Radix Et Rhizoma Rhei (*Da Huang*), Cortex Phellodendri (*Huang Bai*), Rhizoma Curcumae Longae (*Jiang Huang*), and Radix Angelicae (*Bai Zhi*), 500g @, Rhizoma Atractylodis (*Cang Zhu*), Cortex Magnoliae Officinalis (*Hou Po*), and Radix Glycyrrhizae (*Gan Cao*), 200g @, Radix Trichosanthis Kirlowii (*Hua Fen*), 1000g. Grind (the above ingredients) into a fine powder. Mix with warm, boiled water or honey into a paste and apply (to the affected area).

Functions and indications: Clears heat and eliminates dampness, scatters stasis, stops pain, and disperses swelling in the treatment of erysipelas, etc.

(19) *Si Huang San*: Equal parts Radix Et Rhizoma Rhei (*Da Huang*), Cortex Phellodendri (*Huang Bai*), Radix Scutellariae Baicalensis (*Huang Qin*), and Rhizoma Coptidis Chinensis (*Huang Lian*). Grind (the above) into a fine powder. Mix with warm, boiled water or honey and apply to the affected area.

Functions and indications: Disperses inflammation and resolves toxins, disperses swelling and stops pain in the treatment of erysipelas, swelling due to furuncles, folliculitis, etc.

Supplement: *Si Huang Gao*: *Si Huang San*, 20g and petroleum jelly, 80g. Melt the petroleum jelly and mix thoroughly (with the above powdered herbs) to form a paste. (Its) functions and indications are the same as for *Si Huang San*.

(20) *Qing Dai San*: Indigo Naturalis (*Qing Dai*) and Cortex Phellodendri (*Huang Bai*), 20g @, and Gypsum Fibrosum (*Shi Gao*) and Talcum (*Hua Shi*), 40g @. Grind (each ingredient) separately and mix thoroughly. Use cold, boiled water to make into a paste for application.

Functions and indications: Absorbs dampness and stops itching, clears heat and resolves toxins in the treatment of dermatitis due to (allergy to) chemical drugs, eczema, etc.

Qing Dai Gao: *Qing Dai San*, 25g and petroleum jelly, 100g. Melt (the petroleum jelly) and mix together thoroughly. Use externally.

Functions and indications: Disperses inflammation and stops itching, clears heat and resolves toxins in the treatment of eczema and dermatitis *without* secretion of serous fluid

(21) *Sheng Ji Gao*: Powdered Borax (*Peng Sha*), 60g, Borneolum Syntheticum (*Bing Pian*), 60g, Herba Menthae (*Bo He*), 10g, Minium (*Qian Dan*), 30g, zinc oxide 120g, powdered Margarita (*Zhen Zhu*), 10g, phenol 2g, and petroleum jelly 2500g. Mix thoroughly for external use only.

Functions and indications: (Promotes) the generation of (new) tissue and evacuates toxins in the treatment of chronic ulceration of the lower extremities, etc.

(22) *Run Ji Gao*: Radix Angelicae sinensis (*Dang Gui*) and Cera Flava (*Huang La*), 15g @, Radix Lithospermi Seu Arnebiae (*Zi Cao*), 3g, roasted sesame oil (*Xiang You*), 120g. Fry the Radix Angelicae Sinensis and Radix Lithospermi in the sesame oil (until the medicinals are burnt). Remove the dregs and add the Cera Flava. For external application.

Functions and indications: Moistens the skin and stops itching in the treatment of rhagas of the extremities, seborrheic dermatitis, ichthyosis, etc.

(23) *Bai Xie Feng Ding*: Fructus Cnidii Monnieri (*She Chuang Zi*) and Radix Sophorae Flavescentis (*Ku Shen*), 30g @, Cortex Pseudolaricis (*Tu Jing Pi*), 15g, Oleum Menthae (*Bo He You*), 6g, and 75% alcohol 1000 ml. Soak (the ingredients) in the alcohol for one week. (The tincture) is ready when (the ingredients) are strained out. Apply externally.

Functions and indications: Removes dandruff and stops itching in the treatment of seborrheic dermatitis

(24) *Hong Ling Jiu*: Raw Radix Angelicae Sinensis (*Sheng Dang Gui*) and skin of Cortex Cinnamomi (*Rou Gui Pi*), 60g @, Flos Carthami Tinctorii (*Hong Hua*), Rhizoma Desiccata Zingiberis (*Gan Jiang*), and Fructus Zanthoxyli Bungeani (*Chuan Jiao*), 30 g @, Camphora (*Zhang Nao*) and Herba Cum Radice Asari Seiboldi (*Xi Xin*), 15g @, and 95% alcohol 1000 ml. Soak (the above ingredients in the alcohol) for one week before straining. For external use (only).

Functions and indications: Warms the channels, activates the blood, and scatters cold in the treatment of frostbite, scleroderma, etc.

(25) *Zhi Yang Ding*: Fructus Cnidii Monnieri (*She Chuang Zi*) and Radix Stemonae (*Bai Bu*), 25g @. Soak in 50% alcohol 100 ml for 24 hours. Strain the dregs and apply externally.

Functions and indications: Stops itching and kills parasites in the treatment of neurodermatitis, pruritus, prurigo, etc. nodularis, and pediculosis

(26) *Yu Lu San*: Grind into a fine powder Folium Hibisci (*Mu Fu Rong Ye*). Mix with warm, boiled water or honey before applying.

Functions and indications: Clears heat and resolves toxins, cools the blood and disperses swelling in the treatment of erysipelas, etc.

(27) *Gan Cao You*: Radix Glycyrrhizae (*Gan Cao*), 35g and roasted sesame oil (*Xiang You*), 500g. Soak the Radix Glycyrrhizae in the sesame oil for 24 hours before frying it to a dark brown color. Strain the dregs and apply externally.

Functions and indications: Moistens dryness and prevents rhagas in the treatment of rhagas of the hands and feet, progressive metacarpophalangeal keratoderma, etc.

(28) *San Huang Xi Ji*: Equal parts Radix Et Rhizoma Rhei (*Da Huang*), Cortex Phellodendri (*Huang Bai*), Radix Scutellariae Baicalensis (*Huang Qin*), and Radix Sophorae Flavescentis (*Ku Shen*). Grind into a fine powder. Mix 10 ml of this medicinal powder with distilled water 100 ml and carbolic acid, 1 ml. For external application (only).

Functions and indications: Clears heat and facilitates astringency, stops itching and disperses inflammation in the treatment of dermatitis due to chemical (allergy), eczema, folliculitis, etc.

(29) *Dian Dao San Xi Ji*: Powdered Radix Et Rhizoma Rhei (*Da Huang Fen*) and powdered Sulphur (*Liu Huang Fen*), 75g @. Add concentrated limestone water (*Shi Tan Shui*) up to 1000 ml. For external use.

Functions and indications: Clears heat and resolves toxins, stops itching and kills parasites in the treatment of acne, brandy nose, etc.

(30) *Ku Shen Tang*: Radix Sophorae Flavescentis (*Ku Shen*) and Flos Chrysanthemi Morifolii (*Ju Hua*), 60g @, Fructus Cnidii Monnieri (*She Chuang Zi*) and Flos Lonicerae Japonicae (*Jin Yin Hua*), 30g @, Radix Angelicae (*Bai Zhi*), Cortex Phellodendri (*Huang Bai*), Fructus Kochiae (*Di Fu Zi*) and Rhizoma Acori Graminei (*Shi Chang Pu*), 15g @. Wash and steam (the affected area) with the medicated decoction.

Functions and indications: Dispels wind and eliminates dampness, kills parasites and stops itching in the treatment of eczema of the hip, tinea of the hands and feet, etc.

(31) *Yin Xie Bing Yu Ji*: Alum (*Ku Fan*) and Fructus Zanthoxyli Bungeani (*Chuan Jiao*), 120g @, Mirabilitum (*Po Xiao*), 500g, Flos Chrysanthemi Indici (*Ye Ju Hua*), 250g. Boil in 10 k of water. Wash and bath the affected area with the juice after straining.

Functions and indications: Stops itching and kills parasites in the treatment of keratolysis, psoriasis, etc.

(32) *Yan Xun Liao Fa* **(Fumigation Therapy):** Cortex Radicis Dictamni

(*Bai Xian Pi*), Fructus Carpesii Abrotanoidis (*He Shi*), Colophonium (*Song Xiang*), 60g @, Rhizoma Atractylodis (*Cang Zhu*), Radix Sophorae Flavescentis (*Ku Shen*), and Cortex Phellodendri (*Huang Bai*), 45g @, Semen Hydnocarpi (*Da Feng Zi*), 150g, and Galla Rhi Chinensis (*Wu Bei Zi*), 75g. Grind the above herbs into a fine powder. Roll 7g of the above powder in two pieces of tissue paper. Ignite and fumigate the affected area. Each (treatment) should last 10-15 minutes.

Functions and indications: Stops itching and kills parasites in the treatment of neuroderma, chronic eczema, tinea of the hands and feet, etc.

(33) *Fu Fang Ku Shen Fen*: Powdered Gypsum Fibrosum (*Shi Gao Fen*), 500g, powdered Radix Sophorae Flavescentis (*Ku Shen Fen*), 120g, Camphora (*Zhang Nao*) and powdered Semen Phaseoli Munginis (*Lu Dou Fen*), 30g @, Borneol (*Bing Pian*), 50g. Grind the Gypsum with water first and dry it in the shade before mixing thoroughly with the other powders.

Functions and indications: Disperses inflammation and stops itching in the treatment of diaper rash, summertime dermatitis, etc.

(34) *Hong Teng You Gao*: Indigo Naturalis (*Qing Dai*), Herba Portulacae (*Ma Chi Xian*), Acacia Catechu (*Er Cha*), Borneol (*Bing Pian*), and Cortex Phellodendri (*Huang Bai*), 100g @, Galla Rhi Chinensis (*Wu Bei Zi*), 50g, petroleum jelly, 1000g. Grind the above medicinals, except the petroleum jelly, into a fine powder. Mix with the petroleum jelly individually. When (all the ingredients) have been thoroughly mixed, the paste is ready (for use).

Functions and indications: Promotes astringency, stops itching, and disperses inflammation in the treatment of diaper rash, etc.

(35) *Hua Bang Jie Du Tang*: Gypsum Fibrosum (*Shi Gao*), 30g, Rhizoma Cimicifugae (*Sheng Ma*), Fructus Forsythiae Suspensae (*Lian Qiao*), Fructus Arctii (*Niu Bang Zi*), Rhizoma Coptidis Chinensis (*Huang Lian*), Rhizoma Anemarrhenae (*Zhi Mu*), Radix Scrophulariae Ningpoensis (*Yuan Shen*), and Herba Lopthatheri Gracilis (*Dan Zhu Ye*), 10g @. Decoct with water and take.

Functions and indications: Cools the blood, clears heat, and resolves toxins in the treatment of lacquer dermatitis, erysipelas, etc.

(36) *Qing Ying Tang*: Cornu Rhinoceri (*Xi Jiao*), 1g, ground into powder and taken separately, Radix Rehmanniae (*Sheng Di*) and Flos Lonicerae Japonicae (*Jin Yin Hua*), 30g @, Radix Scrophulariae Ningpoensis (*Yuan Shen*), Herba Lopthatheri Gracilis (*Dan Zhu Ye*), and Fructus Forsythiae Suspensae (*Lian Qiao*), 15g @, Rhizoma Coptidis Chinensis (*Huang Lian*), Sclerotium Poriae Cocoris (*Fu Ling*), and Tuber Ophiopogonis Japonicae (*Mai Dong*), 10g @. Decoct with water and take.

Functions and indications: Clears the *ying* phase or level and resolves toxins, discharges heat and nourishes yin in the treatment of chemically (induced) allergic dermatitis, etc.

(37) *Er Miao Wan*: Rhizoma Atractylodis (*Cang Zhu*), 60g, soaked in rice wash water and Cortex Phellodendri (*Huang Bai*), 40g, fried with wine. Grind (the above two ingredients) into a fine powder and pill with wheat flour paste into the size of Chinese parasol tree seeds. Take the pills orally.

Functions and indications: Clears heat and transforms dampness in the treatment of eczema, etc.

(38) *Si Wu Tang*: Radix Coquitus Rehmanniae (*Shu Di*), 30g, Radix Angelicae Sinensis (*Dang Gui*), 15g, Radix Albus Paeoniae Lactiflorae (*Bai Shao*), 12g, and Radix Ligustici Wallichii (*Chuan Xiong*), 9g. Decoct with water and take.

Functions and indications: Nourishes and supplements the blood in the treatment of chronic eczema, etc.

(39) *Long Dan Xie Gan Tang*: Radix Gentianae Scabrae (*Long Dan Cao*) and Radix Rehmanniae (*Sheng Di*), 15g @, Rhizoma Alismatis (*Ze Xie*), Semen Plantaginis (*Che Qian Zi*), and Radix Scutellariae Baicalensis (*Huang Qin*), 12g @, Fructus Gardeniae Jasminoidis (*Shan Zhi Zi*), Caulis Akebiae Mutong (*Mu Tong*), Radix Angelicae Sinensis (*Dang Gui*), and Radix Bupleuri (*Chai Hu*), 9g @, and Radix Glycyrrhizae (*Gan Cao*), 3g. Decoct with water and take.

Functions and indications: Clears liver fire and disinhibits damp heat in the treatment of herpes zoster, auricular eczema, scrotal pruritus, pruritus vulvae, etc.

(40) *Pi Zhi Gao*: Indigo Naturalis (*Qing Dai*) and Cortex Phellodendri (*Huang Bai*), 20g @, and prepared Gypsum Fibrosum (*Duan Shi Gao*), 200g. Grind into a fine powder and mix with sesame oil (*Ma You*). Apply externally.

Functions and indications: Disperses inflammation and stops itching in the treatment of auricular eczema, eczema of the hip, keratosis follicularis, etc.

(41) *Huang Lian Jie Du Tang*: Rhizoma Coptidis Chinensis (*Huang Lian*), 15g, Radix Scutellariae Baicalensis (*Huang Qin*) and Cortex Phellodendri (*Huang Bai*), 12g @, and Fructus Gardeniae Jasminoidis (*Shan Zhi Zi*), 9g. Decoct with water and take.

Functions and indications: Discharges heat (through) bitter, cold (properties), clears fire and resolves toxins in the treatment of pyoderma, etc.

(42) *Bu Ji Xiao Du Yin*: Radix Isatidis Seu Baphicacanthi (*Ban Lan Gen*), 30g, Radix Scutellariae Baicalensis (*Huang Qin*), Rhizoma Coptidis Chinensis (*Huang Lian*), and Fructus Forsythiae Suspensae (*Lian Qiao*), 12g @, Radix Scrophulariae Ningpoensis (*Yuan Shen*), 15g, Radix Glycyrrhizae (*Gan Cao*), Fructus Arctii (*Niu Bang Zi*), Radix Platycodi Grandiflori (*Jie Gen*), and Rhizoma Cimicifugae (*Sheng Ma*), 9g @, Herba Menthae (*Bo He*) and Bombyx Batryticatus (*Jiang Can*), 6g @, Pericarpium Citri Reticulatae (*Chen Pi*) and Fructificatio Lasiospherae (*Ma Bo*), 3g @, and Radix Bupleuri (*Chai Hu*) 5g. Decoct with water and take.

Functions and indications: Clears heat, resolves toxins, and disperses swelling in the treatment of erysipelas of the facial area, etc.

(43) *Chai Hu Qing Gan Tang*: Radix Rehmanniae (*Sheng Di*), 25g, Radix Angelicae Sinensis (*Dang Gui*), Radix Albus Paeoniae Lactiflorae (*Bai Shao*), Radix Bupleuri (*Chai Hu*), Radix Scutellariae Baicalensis (*Huang Qin*), Fructus Gardeniae Jasminoidis (*Shan Zhi Zi*), Radix Trichosanthis Kirlowii (*Hua Fen*), Radix Ledebouriellae Sesloidis (*Fang Feng*), Fructus Arctii (*Niu Bang Zi*), Fructus Forsythiae Suspensae (*Lian Qiao*), and Radix Glycyrrhizae (*Gan Cao*), 10g @, and Radix Ligustici Wallichii (*Chuan Xiong*), 5g. Decoct with water and take.

Functions and indications: Clears the liver and resolves depression, facilitates antisepsis and resolves toxins in the treatment of erysipelas of the waist and costal regions, etc.

(44) *Wu Sheng Tang*: Flos Lonicerae Japonicae (*Jin Yin Hua*) and Herba Violae Yedoensis (*Zi Hua Di Ding*), 30g @, Sclerotium Poriae Cocoris (*Fu Ling*), Radix Achyranthis Bidentatae (*Niu Xi*), and Semen Plantaginis (*Che Qian Zi*), 12g @. Decoct with water and take.

Functions and indications: Clears heat and eliminates dampness in the treatment of erysipelas of the lower extremities, etc.

(45) *Lu Yao Gao*: Sesame oil (*Ma You*) and pig's bile (*Zhu Dan Ye*) 100g @, Semen Ricini Communis (*Bi Ma Zi*), 49 pcs., Aerugo (*Tong Lu*), 60g, Colophonium (*Song Xiang*), 250g. Heat the sesame oil in a clay pot. Then add the mashed Semen Ricini Communis and (cook) until it is burnt. Strain the dregs. Add the Colophonium and melt it in the well boiled oil. Next, add the bile and Aerugo and mix thoroughly with the oil. Wash this mixture in water 100 times. The more one washes, the greener (the mixture) will become. Re-melt by steaming before application.

Functions and indications: Evacuates toxins and disperses inflammation in the treatment of suppurative penetrating perifolliculitis of the head, etc.

(46) *Liu Wei Di Huang Wan*: Radix Coquitus Rehmanniae (*Shu Di*), 240g, Fructus Corni Officinalis (*Shan Zhu Yu*) and Radix Dioscoreae Oppositae (*Shan Yao*), 120g @, Cortex Radicis Moutan (*Dan Pi*), Sclerotium Poriae Cocoris (*Fu Ling*), and Rhizoma Alismatis (*Ze xie*), 90g @. Grind the above herbs into a fine powder and pill the size of Chinese parasol tree seeds. Take 15g each time, 2 times per day with a light salt solution.

Functions and indications: Enriches and nourishes the kidney yin in the treatment of sclerotic erythema, lupus erythematosus, etc.

(47) **Modified** *Shui Jing Gao*: Soak glutinous rice in 20% sodium hydroxide for 24 hours. Grind (the rice) for use. When applied externally, (be sure that) the normal (area) of the skin is well protected. As soon as there is a burning sensation (around the affected area), the treatment should be aborted by removing the powdered rice.

Functions and indications: Softens the hard by erosion in the treatment of clavus or corns, warts on the soles, etc.

Appendix II: Glossary

Acneiform eruptions: lesions resembling acne but lacking comedones, and usually beginning suddenly

Annular lesions: circles made of individual lesions

Atrophy: thinning and wrinkling of the skin resembling cigarette paper

Blister: a vesicle more than 5 mm in diameter

Callosity: a superficial, circumscribed area of hyperkeratosis at a site of repeated trauma

Clavus: a corn

Corn: a painful, conical hyperkeratosis found principally over the toe joints and between the toes

Cyst: an elevated lesion containing fluid or viscous material appearing as a papule or nodule

Epidermolysis: the breakdown of the epidermis

Erosion: loss of part or all of the epidermis

Erythema: redness of the skin

Excoriation: a linear or hollowed out, crusted area, caused by scratching, rubbing, or picking

Exfoliation: the shedding or peeling of the superficial layers of the skin

Furfuraceous: covered with dandruff; scurfy

Hyperkeratosis: overgrowth of the horny layer of the skin

Irregular groupings: lesions occurring in no distinct pattern

Keloid: a smooth overgrowth of fibroblastic tissue that arises in an area of injury or occasionally spontaneously

Lichenification: thickening of the skin with accentuation of skin markings

Macule: a flat, discolored spot of varied size and shape, less than 10 mm in diameter

Maculopapule: slightly elevated macules

Mycosis: any infection caused by a fungus

Nodule: a palpable, solid lesion, more than 5 or 10 mm in diameter, that may or may not be elevated

Papule: a solid, elevated lesion usually less than 10 mm in diameter

Plaque: a group of confluent papules

Pruritus: itching

Purpura: hemorrhage into the skin

Purulent: containing pus

Pustule: a superficial, elevated lesion containing pus

Pyoderma: a pustular condition of the skin

Pyogenic: pus-forming

Retiform grouping: lesions forming a network

Rhagas (pl. rhagades): a fissure or cleavage of the epidermis extending into the dermis

Scabs: Dried serum, blood, or pus

Scales: heaped-up particles of horny epithelium

Scar: the result of healing after destruction of some of the dermis

Sclerosis: induration of an area of skin from underlying interstitial inflammation

Serpiginous grouping: lesions occurring in wavy lines

Suppurate: to form pus

Telangiectasia: dilation of superficial blood vessels

Ulcer: loss of epidermis and at least part of the dermis

Vegetation: an elevated, irregular growth

Vesicle: A circumscribed, elevated lesion less than 5 mm in diameter, that contains serous fluid

Wheal: a transient, elevated lesion caused by local edema

Zosteriform grouping: lesions occurring in broad bands

dermatitis, vesicular 111, 113
dermatitis, white clipping 129
dermatomyositis 117
dermatophytids 60
dermatosis due to lacquer allergy 3
dermographism 91
desquamation 8, 23, 26, 51, 56, 108, 146
desquamation, furfuraceous 108
diabetes 93
diagnosis, four methods of 3
diaper rash 19, 157
diarrhea 33, 61
die wa xian 59
dietary medicine 1
diffuse infiltration 84
dihydroxyphenylalanine 123
ding ji 14
dog bite 45
dong chuang 100
dong zhu 100
dryness 5-8, 11, 54, 56, 67, 91-93, 103,
  104, 109, 129, 130, 134, 137, 151, 156
dryness, internal 7, 8
dung wu xue xi chong wei ao pi yan 77
duo xing hong ban 106

E

e kou chuang 61
e zhua feng 57
ears 25, 129
eczema 3, 10, 11, 15, 22-27, 29, 30, 32,
  37, 45, 65, 150, 151, 154, 156,
  157-159
eczema around the hip 27
eczema, aural 25
eczema, chronic 24
eczema, infantile 3, 10, 26, 31, 32, 151
eczema of the hand 29
eczema, periumbilical 30
eczema, scrotal 28
eczema, subacute 23, 24
edema, local 33, 162
edema, massive, puffy 41

edema, substantial facial 117
eight principles 3
elbows and knees, lateral sides of 103
emaciation 120
endocrine system, disorders of the 93,
  123
entangled melon vine 120
epidermis, thickening of the horny layer of
  98
Entering the Gate of Medicine 99
er bu shi zheng 25
er zhen 16
erysipelas 41, 153-155, 157, 159, 160
erythema due to irritation by fire 147
erythema, epidermolytic 21
erythema induratum 65
erythema, light purple 117
erythema, moist 18
erythema, multiform 3, 21
erythema, nodular 12, 46, 104
erythema, reticular 147
erythema, scarlatina-like 21
erythema, urticaria-like 21
Essential Points of Wai Ke 1
exfoliation, epidermal 26
extracts 14
eyebrow arch 129
eyebrows 84, 135
eyelids 20, 70, 117

F

fa ji chuang 42
fall 35, 37, 44, 50, 55, 93, 103, 105,
  106, 109, 119, 125, 130, 135, 139
fats and carbohydrates, over-eating 131
Favus fungus 49
fei chuang 49
fei cuo chuang 99
fei zi 99
fen du kuai 76
fen ji 14
ferruginous microsporia 50
fetal toxins 31, 44

inflammation 4, 13-15, 17, 18, 41, 49, 85, 153, 154, 156, 157, 159, 160, 162
inguinal grooves 63
insect sting 8
insomnia 20
internal organs, hyperactivity of fire in 8
itchiness, extreme 6
itchiness, variable 37
itching condition 93
itching, intolerable 35, 37, 53
itching, unpredictable bouts of 30

J

jaundice 93
ji chuang 30, 42, 145
ji di xi bao ai 141
ji yan 97, 117
ji yi 1
jia xian 57
jie 1, 17, 20, 38, 42, 44, 62, 63, 78, 79, 85, 92, 94, 104, 108, 112, 122, 149-151, 157, 159
jie chuang 78
jie zhong 38
jin yin chuang 22, 25, 27, 28, 30, 31
jiu zha bi 132
jock itch 52
joints, soreness and pain of 120
jun lie chuang 98

K

keloids 42, 141
keratosis, perifollicular 138
knees, lateral sides of elbows and 103
Kolmer's serum tests 89
kou qiang nian mo nien zhu jun bin e kou chuang 61
kou shui xing pi yan 18

L

labial area, irritation of 18
lagophthalmos 83
lassitude, general 115, 146
lei li xing pi fu jie he 63
leprosy 2, 83, 84
leprotic epidemic area 84
lesion, cat's eye 106
lesion, fetal astringency 31
lesion, fire mark 147
lesion, flaming red 111
lesion, girdle-like 119
lesion, goat's beard 40
lesion, guttate 119
lesion, infiltrative 28
lesion, lice 80
lesion, miliaria acne 99
lesion, mole cricket 44
lesion, obesity 49
lesion, swallow's nest 40
lesion, tertiary mucosal 88
lesion, tertiary neurological 88
lesion, tertiary ocular 88
lesion, umbilical 30
lesion, yellow water 37
leukocytes 115
leukoderma 5, 58, 83
leukorrhea 93
li hei 125
li qing pi yan 146
Li Yan 99
li yang feng 58
lian chuang 31, 45
lice 8, 75, 80
lichenification 8, 23, 27, 28, 161
lie li 63
lip, upper 40
liver and heart fire 41
liver and kidneys, insufficiency of 5
liver and spleen, enlargement of 89, 115
liver channel, damp heat in 28
locomotive impairment 117
lou gu jie 44

lumbar soreness 6, 115
lump, frozen 100
lymph nodes, enlarged 37, 41, 89
lymph nodes, swelling and pain of 121
lungs and stomach, ascent of wind heat
   from the 108

M

ma feng 83
macula and scabs, itchy 103
macula lutea 126
macules, oval 108
maculopapules 19
*mai xing pan zhuang hong ban xing lang
   chuang* 116
malaise 7, 46, 115, 120
man xing xia tui kuei yang 45
mao nong yan 39
mao nong zhou wei jiao hua bin 138
mao yan chuang 106
medicine, internal 1
mei du 87
melanocytes 123
melanosis, skin 125
menstruation, abnormal 115
menstruation, irregular 6, 120
mental confusion 20
metastasis 142
mian you feng 129
micrococcus pyogenes 42
miliaria 37, 99
miliaria acne lesion 99
miliaria rubra 99
mites 34, 78, 79
moniliasis 57
mosquitos 34, 75
moxibustion 15, 67
mu zi xian 109
myalgia 121
Mycobacterium leprae 83-85
mycosal infection 51

N

nail, ashy 57
nausea 6, 7, 121, 146
neck 20, 23, 31, 38, 39, 42, 63, 70, 91,
   99, 117, 125, 126, 129, 146
necrosis 17, 45
needles, body 16
needles, plum blossom 16
nephritis 38, 79, 115
nerves, peripheral 73, 83
nervous dysfunction 123
nervus peroneus communis 83
nervus ulnaris 83
neurodermatitis 11, 15, 16, 91, 94, 155
neurological skin disorders 91
nipple, cracked 26
nipple, cracked, complicated by eczema
   26
nipple feels itchy 26
nipple, rat's 70
nipple wind 26
niu pi xian 91
nodulations, dark red 8
nodulations, numerous 5
nodulations, subcutaneous 8
nong bao chuang 37
nong cao chuang 37
*nong zhong chuang chu xing tou bu mao
nang zhou wei yan* 44
nose, hammer 132
nu yin kuei yang 46

O

odor, body 133
odor like mouse urine 49
ointments 14
ointments, oil-based 14
over-eating fats and carbohydrates 131

P

pain 3, 8, 11, 13, 14, 17, 21, 33, 38, 40, 41, 45, 46, 53, 54, 56, 65, 69, 73, 75, 77, 83, 88, 98, 105, 107, 111, 116, 118, 120, 121, 139, 141, 148, 153, 154
pain, localized inflammation and 41
pain, paroxysms of severe 45
panniculitis 12, 120, 152
papules 5-8, 17, 19, 23, 27, 30-31, 39, 40, 43, 51, 67, 68, 75-77, 79, 83, 87, 91, 99, 101, 103, 106, 113, 131, 132, 138, 162
papules, densely spotted 99
papules, fecal toxin 76
papules, inflammatory, with a hair at the center 40
papules, reddish 19
papules, scattered, puffy 76
papulo-vesicles the size of pin heads 99
paralysis, facial 83
parasites 23, 33, 46, 75, 155-157
parasites, intestinal 23, 33
pastes 13
patches, creamy white 61
pei lei 33
pemphigus 111, 112
pemphigus, common 111
pemphigus foliaceous 111
pemphigus vegetans 112
penicillin 21
perineum 52, 91, 133
pestilential qi, epidemic 83
phalanges, absorption of 83
phenobarbital 21
pi fu hei bian bing 125
pi ji yan 117
pigment, disappearance of 123
pigment sedimentation 4, 23, 35
pigment sedimentation with a distinct border 23
pigmentation, reticular 147
pinworm 93
pityriasis rosacea 109

pityriasis simplex 108
placenta 87
plaques, circular 50, 51
plaques, ivory colored, small 119
plaques with distinctive borders 103
pleurisy 115
pneumonia 72, 115
pneumonia, interstitial 115
powders 14, 42, 81, 134, 157
Prescriptions for Emergency 1
prickly heat 99
private parts, erosion of 46
protracted course 7, 43, 45
pruritus 16, 22, 93, 94, 151, 155, 158, 162
pruritus, perianal 93, 94
pruritus, scrotal 93, 158
pruritus, senile 93
pruritus, systemic 93, 94
pruritus vulvae 93, 94, 158
psoriasis 9, 11, 103, 104, 149, 156
puberty 131
pudenda 39
pus, discharge of 4, 31, 44
pus, drainage of 13
pus nest lesion 37
pus, purulent 31
pustulae have spread widely 38
pustules 4, 7, 8, 11, 13, 19, 23, 30, 40, 51, 55, 70, 75, 113
pustules, pinhead-like 19
pustulosis 37
pyoderma 80, 150, 151, 159, 162

Q

qi bu shi zheng 30
Qi De-zhi 2
Qi Kun 30
qi xing pi yan 19
qian ma zheng 33, 34
qian ri chuang 67
que ban 124

R

rash, delicate skin 34
rash, lacquer 19
re qi chuang 72
redness 8, 11, 38, 99, 105, 117, 135, 161
retroauricular area 25
Revealing the Mystery of Wai Ke 14, 15, 19, 27, 45, 51, 55
rhagas 5, 8, 56, 155, 156, 162
rou ci 97
ru tou feng 26
ru tou jun lie xing shi zheng 26

S

sacrum 91, 113
scab, crust-like 49
scabies 2, 3, 8, 15, 78
scabs 5, 6, 23, 25, 28, 31, 37, 49, 51, 80, 93, 102, 103, 111, 112, 121, 130, 162
scabs, grayish brown 28
scaling 4, 5, 9, 22, 28, 51, 54, 55, 109, 112, 117, 121, 135, 137, 139
scaling, adhesive 117
scaling, brown or dark, fishlike 137
scalp 39, 49, 50, 103, 119, 129, 134
scarring 131
scars, atrophic 44
scars, bundle-like 63
Schistoma japonica 77
Schistosoma cercariae flukes 77
schistosomiasis 77
scleroderma 10, 118, 150, 155
scratch marks 102
scrofula 63
scrofular cutaneous tuberculosis 63
scrotum 23, 28, 91
sebaceous glands, hypersecretion of 129
sensations of heat and pain 75
serous fluid, discharge of 7, 37

serum reactivity 89
sex hormones 139
sexual function, impeded 120
shan lou 65
she chuan chuang 73
she pi xian 137
shen jing xing pi yan 91
shen nang feng 28
shi bin 80
shi chuang 80
shi fu 15
shi yi 1
shi zheng 25-27, 29, 30
shoe size, inappropriate 97
shou bu shi zheng 29
shou xian 53
shou yi 1
shou zu jun lie 98
shoulder 113, 117
shu jie 38
shu ru 70
shui fen ji 14
shui ji chuang 145
skin appendages, disorders of 129
skin, atrophy of due to old age 93
skin disease, dyschromatic 123
skin disease, erythematous scaly 103
skin disease, nodular painful 12
skin disease, sitting board 27
skin disorders, neurological 91
skin, dry 4, 8, 83, 129
skin, hypertrophic 27
skin, infirmity of the striae of 17
skin melanosis 125
skin, striae of the 15, 17
skin tumors 141
skin, wrinkled 89
sleeping pills 21
song pi xian 103
sores, goose mouth 61
sores, hot qi 72
sores, snake-like cluster 73
sores, thousand day 67
spermatorrhea 6

Formula Index

P

Pei Pa Qing Fei Yin 131
Pi Zhi Gao 26, 27, 41, 108, 138, 159
Pian Zhi Gao 98

Q

Qian Chui Gao 13, 39, 152
Qing Dai Gao 14, 22, 24, 26, 77, 78, 80, 106, 107, 114, 116, 147, 154
Qing Dai San 14, 20, 32, 38, 113, 154
Qing Hao Yi Ren Tang 10, 150
Qing Huo Yi Ren Tang 102
Qing Shu Tang 10, 39, 150
Qing Ying Tang 22, 158
Qu Feng Di Huang Wan 54

R

Run Fu Tang 11, 93, 137, 151
Run Ji Gao 14, 32, 99, 130, 137-139, 154

S

San Huang Wan 43
San Huang Xi Ji 15, 18, 22, 24, 40, 61, 75, 77, 78, 102, 110, 113, 114, 132, 148, 156
San Xian Dan 89, 133
San Xian Dan He Ji 89
Shao Feng Wan 85
Shen Ying Yang Zhen Dan 135
Sheng Di Yin Hua Tang 11, 20, 152
Sheng Ji Gao 14, 46, 47, 86, 90, 101, 154
Sheng Ji San 31, 66
Shui Jing Gao 71, 98, 160
Si Huang Gao 14, 154
Si Huang San 14, 39, 40, 42, 113, 114, 153, 154
Si Wu Tang 24, 133, 152, 158

T

Ta Yang Tang 47
Tai Yi Gao 13, 39, 153
Tu Fu Ling He Ji 90

W

Wu Hu Dan 142
Wu Wei Xiao Du Yin 11, 39, 130, 151

X

Xi Xian Wan 124
Xiao Feng Dao Che Tang 32
Xiao Feng San 9, 17, 24, 149
Xin Yi Qing Fei Yin 72
Xu You Gao 51

Y

Yang He Tang 10, 120, 150
Yin Xie Bing Yu Ji 15, 104, 156
Yin Xin Wu You San 80
Yu Lu San 14, 42, 106, 155
Yu Ping Feng San 9, 34, 149

Z

Zhi Yang Ding 14, 35, 76, 92, 94, 95, 102, 155

OTHER BOOKS ON CHINESE MEDICINE
AVAILABLE FROM
BLUE POPPY PRESS

1775 Linden Ave
Boulder, CO 80304
For ordering 1-800-487-9296
PH. 303\442-0796 FAX 303\447-0740

PMS: Its Cause, Diagnosis & Treatment According to Traditional Chinese Medicine by Bob Flaws ISBN 0-936185-22-8 $14.95

SOMETHING OLD, SOMETHING NEW; Essays on the TCM Description of Western Herbs, Pharmaceuticals, Vitamins & Minerals by Bob Flaws ISBN 0-936185-21-X $19.95

SCATOLOGY & THE GATE OF LIFE: The Role of the Large Intestine in Immunity, An Integrated Chinese-Western Approach by Bob Flaws ISBN 0-936185-20-1 $12.95

SECOND SPRING: A Guide To Healthy Menopause Through Traditional Chinese Medicine by Honora Lee Wolfe ISBN 0-936185-18-X $14.95

MIGRAINES & TRADITIONAL CHINESE MEDICINE: A Layperson's Guide by Bob Flaws ISBN 0-936185-15-5 $11.95

STICKING TO THE POINT: A Rational Methodology for the Step by Step Formulation & Administration of an Acupuncture Treatment by Bob Flaws ISBN 0-936185-17-1 $14.95

ENDOMETRIOSIS & INFERTILITY AND TRADITIONAL CHINESE MEDICINE: A Laywoman's Guide by Bob Flaws ISBN 0-936185-14-7 $9.95

THE BREAST CONNECTION: A Laywoman's Guide to the Treatment of Breast Disease by Chinese Medicine by Honora Lee Wolfe ISBN 0-936185-13-9 $8.95

NINE OUNCES: A Nine Part Program For The Prevention of AIDS in HIV Positive Persons by Bob Flaws ISBN 0-936185-12-0 $9.95

THE TREATMENT OF CANCER BY INTEGRATED

CHINESE-WESTERN
MEDICINE by Zhang Dai-
zhao, trans. by Zhang Ting-liang
ISBN 0-936185-11-2 $16.95

A HANDBOOK OF
TRADITIONAL CHINESE
DERMATOLOGY by Liang
Jian-hui, trans. by Zhang Ting-
liang & Bob Flaws, ISBN 0-
936185-07-4 $14.95

A HANDBOOK OF
TRADITIONAL CHINESE
GYNECOLOGY by Zhejiang
College of TCM, trans. by Zhang
Ting-liang, ISBN 0-936185-06-6
(2nd edit.) $21.95

FREE & EASY: Traditional
Chinese Gynecology for
American Women 2nd Edition,
by Bob Flaws, ISBN 0-936185-
05-8 $15.95

PRINCE WEN HUI'S
COOK: Chinese Dietary
Therapy by Bob Flaws &
Honora Lee Wolfe, ISBN 0-
912111-05-4, $12.95 (Published by
Paradigm Press, Brookline, MA)

THE DAO OF
INCREASING LONGEVITY
AND CONSERVING ONE'S
LIFE by Anna Lin & Bob Flaws,
ISBN 0-936185-24-4 $16.95

FIRE IN THE VALLEY:
The TCM Diagnosis and
Treatment of Vaginal
Diseases by Bob Flaws
ISBN 0-936185-25-2 $16.95

HIGHLIGHTS OF
ANCIENT ACUPUNCTURE
PRESCRIPTIONS trans. by
Honora Lee Wolfe & Rose
Crescenz ISBN 0-936185-23-6
$14.95

ARISAL OF THE CLEAR:
A Simple Guide to Healthy
Eating According to
Traditional Chinese Medicine
by Bob Flaws, ISBN #-936185-
27-9 $8.95

CERVICAL DYSPLASIA &
PROSTATE CANCER:
HPV, A HIDDEN LINK? by
Bob Flaws, ISBN 0-936185-19-8
$23.95

PEDIATRIC BRONCHITIS:
ITS CAUSE, DIAGNOSIS &
TREATMENT
ACCORDING TO
TRADITIONAL CHINESE
MEDICINE trans. by Gao Yu-li
and Bob Flaws, ISBN 0-936185-
26-0 $15.95

AIDS & ITS TREATMENT
ACCORDING TO
TRADITIONAL CHINESE
MEDICINE by Huang Bing-
shan, trans. by Fu-Di & Bob
Flaws, ISBN 0-936185-28-7
$24.95

ACUTE ABDOMINAL
SYNDROMES: Their
Diagnosis & Treatment by
Combined Chinese-Western
Medicine by Alon Marcus, ISBN
0-936185-31-7 $16.95

BEFORE COMPLETION: Essays on the Practice of TCM by Bob Flaws, ISBN 0-936185-32-5, $16.95

MY SISTER, THE MOON: The Diagnosis & Treatment of Menstrual Diseases by Traditional Chinese Medicine by Bob Flaws, ISBN 0-936185-34-1, $24.95

FU QING-ZHU'S GYNECOLOGY trans. by Yang Shou-zhong and Liu Da-wei, ISBN 0-936185-35-X, $21.95

FLESHING OUT THE BONES: The Importance of Case Histories in Chinese Medicine trans. by Charles Chace. ISBN 0-936185-30-9, $18.95

CLASSICAL MOXIBUSTION SKILLS IN CONTEMPORARY CLINICAL PRACTICE by Sung Baek, ISBN 0-936185-16-3 $10.95

THE MEDICAL I CHING: Oracle of the Healer Within by Miki Shima, OMD, ISBN 0-936185-38-4, $19.95

MASTER TONG'S ACUPUNCTURE: An Ancient Lineage for Modern Practice, trans. and commentary by Miriam Lee, OMD, ISBN 0-936185-37-6, $19.95

A HANDBOOK OF TCM UROLOGY & MALE SEXUAL DYSFUNCTION by Anna Lin, OMD, ISBN 0-936185-36-8, $16.95

Li Dong-yuan's TREATISE ON THE SPLEEN & STOMACH, A Translation of the *Pi Wei Lun* by Yang Shou-zhong & Li Jian-yong, ISBN 0-936185-41-4, $21.95

PATH OF PREGNANCY, VOL. I, Gestational Disorders by Bob Flaws, ISBN 0-936185-39-2, $16.95

PATH OF PREGNANCY, VOL. II, Postpartum Diseases by Bob Flaws, ISBN 0-936185-42-2, $18.95

How to Have a HEALTHY PREGNANCY, HEALTHY BIRTH with Traditional Chinese Medicine by Honora Lee Wolfe, ISBN 0-936185-40-6, $9.95

MASTER HUA'S CLASSIC OF THE CENTRAL VISCERA by Hua Tuo, translated by Yang Shou-zhong, ISBN 0-936185-43-0, $21.95

A NEW AMERICAN ACUPUNCTURE: Acupuncture Osteopathy, by Mark Seem, ISBN 0-936185-44-9, $19.95